Vaccination

Everything You Need to Know About Vaccines

(Everything Your Primary Care Physician May Not Say to You About)

Vincent Williams

Published By **Jordan Levy**

Vincent Williams

Vaccination: Everything You Need to Know About Vaccines (Everything Your Primary Care Physician May Not Say to You About)

ISBN   978-0-9959962-3-6

Legal & Disclaimer

Upon using the information contained in this book, you agree to hold harmless the Author from and against any damages, costs, and expenses, including any legal fees potentially resulting from the application of any of the information provided by this guide. This disclaimer applies to any damages or injury caused by the use and application, whether directly or indirectly, of any advice or information presented, whether for breach of contract, tort, negligence, personal injury, criminal intent, or under any other cause of action.

You agree to accept all risks of using the information presented inside this book. You need to consult a professional medical practitioner in order to ensure you are both able and healthy enough to participate in this program.

Table Of Contents

Chapter 1: Vaccines Holy Icon Of Orthodox Medicine

Vaccines are hailed as the answer to Disease Prevention in the modern medical miracle show. Doctor. Richard Moskowitz called vaccination the "Sacrament of Modern Medicine." Vaccines constitute one of the serpents from the caduceus staff of medical science, representing the current icon of hypodermic needles that protect us from the evil occult that lurks in invisible viruses. "Vaccines are one of the great public health achievements of the last couple centuries" Nurse Alison Buttenheim genuflected in the American Journal of Public Health.

It is the accepted belief system. According to the Center for Disease Control confidently states it is "vaccinating each child born in the United Stated with the current childhood immunization schedule could prevent approximately 42,000 deaths and 20 million cases of the disease."

(although the double-uncertainty sounds like an unreliable math).

The threat of epidemics caused by infectious diseases is a common occurrence since the dawn of time or perhaps due to the urbanization of cities around 10,000 years ago. The belief in vaccinations could be a representation of pilgrims submerging an object into "liquors flowing from the remains" of saints who were buried "a presage of inoculation: a tiny dose or drop if applied would communicate some of the original individual's power to withstand evil." (Marina Warner, London Review of Books October. 2nd 2017, 2017). Most likely the safest option, taking into account other treatments from the past.

Prior to the turn of the century, deaths were incredibly high However, death rates had been declining dramatically in countries that were industrialized in the years prior to the year 1800. Britain was able to boast a 90% reduction in deaths of children due to diseases between 1850 to 1945 however, in the U.S. had a 95 percent reduction in deaths due to diphtheria and pertussis as well as measles and scarlet fever prior to mass vaccination.

Doctor. John Snow is called "the father of public health" due to his identification of a specific water fountain located in London that was responsible for 500 deaths due to cholera within 10 days in 1854. In the event that he stopped the water fountain in which the woman cleaned her infant's nappies it stopped the deaths. His research paper that pointed to the cholera outbreak from water that was contaminated was ridiculed in the past five years, as many doctors believed "miasma in the air caused disease." This was coal smog that was fatal in a completely different manner.

Contagious and deadly illnesses have always created a sense of dread in human beings. Ebola fear and panic across America during 2014 demonstrated that a single death can become a cause for alarm by the fear of being a victim and imbalanced media coverage. Medical propaganda has portrayed the decline in deaths due to infections as a win for vaccination, even though modern vaccines were created following the occurrence of rare deaths. Ninety percent or more of deaths due to infections in the western world were eliminated through health initiatives during the 19th century and into the in the early 20th century. Offering safer drinking water, food and drinks, as well as increasing incomes and better cleanliness, bathing, and sanitation minimized the majority of deaths due to diphtheria, scarlet fever, typhus measles, tetanus and pertussis years before the mass vaccination against these illnesses.

Scarlet Fever , a major death hazard, was eradicated without a vaccine. The Journal of Infection Control acknowledged the fact that "the overall contribution of medical innovations to the health revolution is difficult to validate" in a paper from 2001. The article from 1977 in Lancet one of the British medical journal, was much more direct. "There is no evidence that vaccination played a major role in the decline in incidence and mortality" of infectious diseases.

The diptheria vaccine that was first introduced during the 1890's actually boosted deaths, however improved sanitation, nutrition and ventilation have been credited with dramatically reducing the pertussis mortality rate by the year 1930. The first tetanus vaccination that was based on horses' serums was considered to be the primary source of anaphylaxis. It is an severe allergic condition that afflicts the lungs, throat, intestinal tract, and skin during the first decade of the 20th century. The government issued mandatory vaccinations during that time for smallpox-related outbreaks in the local area however, just for adults because the children were considered to be at risk. Residents were forced by armed policemen to ensure they were vaccines, as a lot of people were ill after the vaccination as well as 1 out of 200 people died.

George Bernard Shaw, a participant in the Health Committee of London (more well-known as a writer and playwright) "learned how the credit of vaccination is kept up statistically by diagnosing all the revaccinated cases as pustular eczema, varioloid or what not- anything exept smallpox." The term is "monkeypox" in Africa now since smallpox is "eradicated."

In 1905 in 1905, The Supreme Court decreed that states were able to impose obligatory vaccinations if there were "imminent harm that imperils an entire population" It could be applied equally to everyone without causing undue damage. In 1922, the Supreme Court affirmed regulations that require children to get vaccination against smallpox to be able to go to schools. This decision was inspired by the utilitarian reasoning that was formulated by an 18th-century British social reformer named Jeremy Bentham. The utilitarian doctrine was employed in the court of Justices in 1923 to permit governments to forcefully sterilize individuals that posed a risk to the wellbeing and health of the society to serve their Greater Good. Following the Nazis carried it to an extreme in WWII The Nuremberg Tribunal decided that utilitarianism was an untrue ethic and established the principle of informed consent as the underlying principle of medical experiments that are ethically based. (NVIC.org)

In 1911, the U.S. military made vaccination compulsory for all new recruits in 1911. They also recorded scores of deaths due to vaccines when they boosted the number of vaccines needed from 15-25 following WWI. They caused 30,000 cases of hepatitis from

their vaccine for yellow fever
(vaclib.org/news/vaccinenotflu).

France refused to offer diptheria
vaccinations following it was declared a
disease during Great War, because cases
rose after the introduction of obligatory
vaccination. The Nazis made the French to
get vaccinated after they defeated them in
Blitzkrieg in 1939. Blitzkrieg in 1939. the
rates of diptheria rose dramatically in 1943,
too.

15 of 19 European Union countries have no
vaccines that are mandatory today,
however their incidences of disease are less
than those of Americans which have the
highest amount of obligatory vaccinations.
No other nation has more mandatory
vaccines. 11 thousand infants born each per
day receive 15-19 doses of vaccination
starting from birth until 18 months to
prevent the 11 common childhood illnesses.
The recommended schedule of 60 vaccines
before the age of preschool is required for

entry and recommendations for annual influenza vaccines each year beginning by giving them to pregnant mothers. The vaccines do not improve overall health since our children's results in health are among the lowest of industrialized countries.

The deterioration in public health within the U.S. to third world standards poses a higher risk than those who are not vaccinated group of exemptions. Instead, the medical industry/government/financial fraternity plans for constructing infrastructure to deliver ten new vaccines now in the development pipeline, with dozens of new genetically modified vaccines in the wings. The company estimates that the market will be worth $100 billion before 2025.

The Wall Street Journal quoted an industry opinion that vaccinations "will be a growing source of revenue to take over older blockbusters that are slated to lose protection from patents. The sales of vaccines are increasing more quickly than prescription drugs and they are protected from generic competition that is costing drug companies billions."

Over 200 brand new vaccines that are in different phases of development and testing in various stages of development, ranging from birth control all the way to cocaine addiction. There are also the latest delivery systems including mosquitoes and genetically engineered fruits.

The Supreme Court ruled again on vaccines in the year 2011, ruling the vaccines to be "unavoidably unsafe", yet there is no court that has jurisdiction on the safety of vaccines. Government regulatory agencies alone have the power to decide if products have been found to be "unreasonably unsafe" for the general public. The government has used this power only sparingly.

It was the National Vaccine Program Office, (NVPO) was deeply concerned about the fact that "adult vaccination rates remain low in the United States." The NVPO wants to reach the targets that are set out by Healthy People 2020 of Health and Human Services. The other medical organizations of the government planned to get parents, health professionals and teachers of the need to "recognize vaccines as a means of mobilizing the body's natural defense." They provide research who "pursue new approaches to vaccine administration more aggressively", as well as "extend the vaccine-delivery service to new populations of adolescents and adults." Medical professionals were urged to promote the belief that vaccinations are standard of conduct in the society. Physicians who disagree "are subject to the harshest scrutiny and punishment", the U.S. National Autism Association advised in 2012.

The National Adult Immunization Plan aggressively target pregnant women, faith group, employers health professionals as well as teachers and parents in order to encourage increased use of vaccines. In the National Vaccine Confidence Working Group set out to boost confidence among consumers and to ensure "optimal use of recommended childhood vaccines in America", specifically targeting "parents whose reluctance, hesitation, concerns or lack of confidence has caused them to question or forego recommended vaccines." They also urged the states to "strengthen" their exemption laws by using coercion instead of convincing for "achieve acceptance" of their objective. Pediatricians get incentives of a few thousands of dollars in exchange for driving greater rates of vaccination for infants and young children.

Following their success with schoolchildren campaign, the adults will be their next target. They will begin with medical professionals as well as childcare staff and teachers. Food service and airline industries are on their list. They have a "long term goal, 100 percent vaccination rates with full government recommendation of vaccines, no exemptions."

(National Vaccine information Center, 2015)

There was no goal for improving the safety of vaccines in order that would increase trust, removal of heavy metals and other harmful ingredients, to conduct long-term studies of safety against placebo-based injections to increase the reporting of physicians of any injuries for the FDA's Vaccine Adverse Events Reporting System (VAERS). It is voluntary to report injuries, but only a tiny fraction of the injuries are recorded. The medical profession is trained to use the procedure only for "serious" injuries including death and disability, as well as hospitalization and when medical intervention is needed. A lot of reports do not contain the essential details needed to identify the risk factor and vaccine lot.

It is believed that through the injection of toxin and virus-laden vaccines in large herds of kids, the ailment illnesses they target will be completely eradicated across the entire populace. Every illness that is covered by mandated vaccines within the U.S. cause few injuries and have near-zero death rates within North America now. The majority of deaths from infectious diseases occur in countries with poorer populations yet effective measures to protect public health are not being utilized in the first and third world regions to favor vaccinations. The cost of vaccines is less than clean drinking water, clean septic systems, and increasing salaries for those living in poverty. The $4.5 billion in the Center for Disease Control spends annually on vaccinations across the U.S. and $30 billion that is spent worldwide leaves health care improvements in a state of begging.

The modern outbreaks of asthma, obesity and diabetes, cancer dementia and heart disease are now world-wide epidemics. Programs to prevent these diseases that are caused by processed eating habits, lifestyles that are sedentary, the stress of high levels of pollution socially deprived society are being starved of the billions of dollars invested in purchasing and advertising vaccinations.

It is not reported that immunologists caution that vaccination-induced immune defense diminishes while combating common childhood diseases creates a deeper T cell defense that is essential for lifetime immunity. They fail to recognize that the vaccine makers are not subject to the safety tests that are conducted using double blind tests against placebos that are genuine. They are snide about epidemiologists that show a strong correlation between neurological and autoimmune disorders through vaccination. They ridicule experts in infectious diseases who say that, after periods of disease-free time due to mass vaccinations, which reduce the natural immune system, much larger outbreaks of more dangerous virus outbreaks will occur.

If they've heard of epigenetics which are changes triggered by the environment to gene expression that may be passed on through generations, they've probably never heard of British epigenetics researcher Dr. Mae Wan Ho's assertion she believes that "vaccines have the potential to generate virulent viruses by recombination and cause autoimmune diseases." They alter the human genome and the intestinal biomes, weakening naturally-generated immunity, and can directly trigger "both short and long term onset of life threatening illnesses affecting millions of people." (Gary Null and Richard Gale, PhD, Vaccinations Dilemna: Not Safe at Every Dose, Global Research, 5/4/2016)

Genetically engineered recombinant virus are also able to escape into the natural environment, and even jump the boundaries between species. Genetic contamination of every vaccination that uses or is grown in human cells from retroviruses prions, proteins, and other viruses, both well-known and unknown are recognized by FDA as well as the CDC. As a result, they have increased the tolerance of contaminants hundred times. They do not consider non- "cancerous cell lines." and urged the elimination of genetically-related contaminants as a "non-binding recommendation."

VACCINE DISSENTERS UNDER SIEGE

Less than 3 percent of parents chose to not having their kids vaccinated for spiritual, religious, or financial motives in California. Even in the richest and most educated counties (where the rates of exemption are at their highest) or those with the lowest and most ineducated (where kids are more likely to be seen by a physician) just less than eight% of all public schools' students were not vaccined. The first three counties have an option to opt-out of the mandatory vaccination schedules for children attending public schools in certain states. The right was repealed in California in the year 2015 and has since been being challenged in the other states which allow exclusions from school.

The Center for Disease Control (CDC) provided an "recipe" for creating "High Vaccine Demand" in 2004 when medical professionals as well as public health officials to "state concern and alarm and predict dire outcomes" of the influenza season. They advised that they label it "very severe" and "deadly." They started expanding their approach to measles and pertussis in the following decade.

The Public Health Law Program (PHLP) created state laws and enforcement procedures. They recommended states to "strengthen the rigor of the application process, frequency of submission and enforcement as strategies to improve vaccination rates" in 2015. If this fails the totalitarian approach are required.

The Disney Measles Mania was in complete chaos, California Senators Barbara Boxer and Diane Feinstein lobbied the state to end any religious or philosophical exemptions. They "oppose even the notion of a medical professional assisting to waive a vaccine requirement unless there is a medical reason" as they urged schools and daycare facilities to "track those families that pledged to get required vaccines after the year begins."

Dr. Robert Pearl, CEO of Permanente Medical Group compared parents who deny their children compulsory vaccination with drunk driving when he was CEO. The attack was coordinated against schoolchildren who were exempted as well as their parents on the media, healthcare platforms, and legislative venues. This is the same as public talking points that were free and unsubstantiated statements were reiterated by doctors and journalists. In the majority of cases, citizens and parents believe it to be an unquestioned truth up until the time their children get injured by vaccinations. Media outlets translate the "public health" officials who are apologists for those from Center for Disease Control and medical associations that dismiss false studies to be "scientific".

Parents are outraged by the fact at the thought that other parents were putting their kids at risk. "This doesn't have to do with your individual beliefs. Santa Claus is a personal conviction. We have vaccinated our family because we have faith in the science." Anne Janks of Oakland made a scene in an story headlined "Vaccine Shy Parents. (San Francisco Chronicle 2/2/15)

"Some people are just incredibly selfish." Dr. James Cherry, a pediatric health specialist from UCLA has spoken out. (Associated Press, 1/23/15) Dr. Cherry blamed the latest

Disneyland measles outbreak to parents who refuse the MMR vaccine to their kids in the school years despite health officials never being able to identify the infector's source. They "anti-science stubbornness has proven that it's a small world after all." The Los Angeles Times quipped in an editorial.

The Dr. Tracy Lieu of Kaiser Permanente stated that "there are clear proofs that having many personal beliefs that are not embraced by communities is linked to the risk of having measles or whooping cough outbreaks."(Marin Independent Journal 1/18/2015) Dr. Lieu was principal researcher in a study of kids who were not vaccinated, that was published in the January. 2015 issue of the Pediatrics journal.

A few weeks later, Three weeks after the Sacramento Bee reported a pertussis outbreak within Elk Grove, California at levels five times more than the other schools within the county. Elk Grove schools were able to get less than 2% of exemptions, 10-to-20 times less than "crazy clusters of exemptors" at other schools. "It's not correct to only pin the pertussis outbreak on people who are unvaccinated." Mark Sawyer, a pediatric physician who is a member of the CDC immunizations practice committee, admitted. It seems he did not read the memo with talking points.

The Marin Immunization Coalition is "a group of local physicians, nurses, teachers, parents and residents of Marin involved in increasing local immunization rates." Co-chairs of the Coalition published an opinion piece titled It's Time to Stop Debating over children's Vaccinations! (Marin Independent Journal, 6/1/15) One is also a participant in the Immunization Workgroup of the National Association of City and County Health Officials. It's a planned agenda. However, the title says the whole thing. "

The opinion of the group was a mix-up of a variety of claims, without any evidence that blamed the resistance to vaccinations to mandatory vaccinations on "visible, albeit ignorant advocates, painful erroneous anecdotes and willful fraud." The authors refer to "Dr. Bob" Sears author of. The Vaccine Book.Dr. Sears affirms in a convincing way to the parents and pediatricians who read the book that he's in favor of vaccination, however the book provides information on positive and negative research in the belief that education based on facts is the most convincing evidence.

The report claimed that he "warns parents not to share their fears with their neighbors, because if too many people avoid the MMR, we'll likely see the diseases increase significantly." I haven't found his recommendation for parents who are exempt from the MMR from the need to "hide in the herd" within the book. It's a suspiciously false argument since the higher rates in "immunization" in countries are connected with a higher rate of illness, according to WHO. World Health Organization.

Journalists, parents, doctors, as well as school officials who believe in the government's claims that vaccinations are completely safe and efficient will likely to hold on to the belief. They'll defend their decision to expose their children to harmful and dangerous toxic substances, in spite of the mounting evidence proving that the vaccine "science" is actually Frankenscience. They aren't trying to prevent them from having that option. They're actively trying to restrict us from exercising our Freedom of Choice.

They do not consider or reject rational, thoughtful investigation of the facts. They are as ignorant as the ones who do refuse to look. News concerning suppressed research appearing in a manner that is systematically ignoring the process of scientific inquiry that is transparent reliable, quantifiable and reproducible proof are not likely to penetrate the wall of their insanity. Cognitive dissonance is a mental method that offers certainty in the midst of a complex and confusing environment yet it imprisons the true adherents in a in self-inforcing data.

There's been a conflict between this camp and parents who think that vaccinations can cause more harm than the potential benefits. The exemptions do not seek to keep other people from getting vaccinated, or exposing their children to these vaccines, however, we could not agree with their decision. It's not so for the Totalitarian Inoculationists. The civil war that seeks to end religious or personal exemptions from obligatory vaccinations in public schools for youngsters has already begun.

Washington and Oregon residents fought back against legislative efforts in the year 2015. California health officials as well as media experts and politicians were in full-on rage using an Disney Measles melee to follow the Mississippi's path in public health. Mississippi tops the list of the infant mortality rate, obesity in childhood as well as diabetes, and rates of vaccination was a perfect model for California lawmakers to prohibit vaccine exemptions.

They compelled Californian parents who educate their children to follow the health policies of Mississippi. The iron buckle that is the Bible Belt doesn't even allow the abolition of religion, let alone philosophical ones. Only Medical Exemptions. "If a medical professional thinks it's wise not to vaccinate, then that will be the gospel." Mississippi Representative John Moore pronounced from his the pulpit of his legislative chambers. This isn't the only metaphor blurring the distinction between state and church in Dixie as well as it's the Golden State.

The parents claim their rights need to be curtailed to protect children that are not vaccination-free. A mere .03 percentage of children have been given medical exemptions to the mandatory vaccinations at school. Most of these children are affected by the mandatory doses of toxic oncology that a greater number of medical toxins are most likely to cause harm or even death for the children. John Hopkins' Hospital Guide for Immunocompromised Patients cautions sufferers to "avoid crowds if possible" as well as close contact with those who have "recently had a live virus vaccination (chicken pox, measles, rubella, nasal spray influenza, polio or smallpox)" due to the fact that the shedding of vaccine viruses is infectious for immune-compromised patients. They don't advise patients against avoiding children who are not vaccinated or adult patients.

Chapter 2: Crazy Clusters Near Whole Foods

An Kaiser Permanente January, 2015 study revealed "clusters of under immunization " (when children don't receive some or all of the recommended shots prior to three years of age) which included levels as high as 23 percentage within "neighborhoods with more families with graduate degrees." A flat vaccination refusal ranged from 5.5-13.5 percentage in the groups in the most wealthy and most educated zip codes within the coastal California areas, as compared to 2.6 percentage in the remainder of California.

The San Francisco Chronicle devoted an article to the "Crazy Clusters"on the 5th of January. "Refusing to give your children the proper number of vaccinations [17 separate injections by the age of 3] shows a lack of courage and responsibility." They acknowledge the fact that "vaccine deniers aren't in need of more education", because graduate degrees can be considered an endpoint in higher education.

It's not clear why higher education creates "anti-scientific beliefs and values." Science, Technology, Engineering and Math (STEM) educational models that are marketed as the best solution to the problem of job security as we move to a world economy America could lead to more conformity to Totalitarian Inoculation than liberal arts.

The tiny percentage of unvaccinated youngsters and their parents are getting blamed for the sporadic cases of vaccination-related ailments that can occur. This seems absurd in the event that vaccines are actually safe and even if "herd immunity" is real. The advocates claim that this has been proved to give security to the community when 70-90 percent of the population is vaccine-vaccinated. The state already has 97.6 percent of California students vaccinated with no restrictions on the exemptions. Schools are only a tiny portion of the population with an aging populace.

It's been a long-running court battle through by the government "health" officials to convince people to follow the recommended schedules for vaccination, particularly because ObamaCare provides the bulk of the vaccines. Doctor. Ruth Haskins, president of the California Medical Association claimed "every resource recommends that pregnant women have the influenza and pertussis vaccines during their pregnancy to protect their unborn child" even though there are no studies on safety performed on pregnant fetuses or including fake ones. Dr. Haskins advised all people who are over 50 years old to receive the shingles vaccine or the majority of them could contract it before the age of 80 due children's chicken pox. If chicken pox or varicella vaccines have only increased number of cases in Korea so why would shingles vaccinations differ. The doctor urged "all people, as long as they don't have a contraindication, [to] have the influenza vaccine." There was no information on what the warnings mean. "I hope seeing the happy faces of people getting vaccinated" in the advertising for public service can encourage more adults to be injected in the future, she said. (Kaiser Health News, 2017,) Except for the fact that they've seen images of adults who are damaged due to vaccines, who are in wheelchairs, or read about five Georgia elderly residents who died in one flu shots.

The herd immunity hypothesis and that of the "antibody-based theory of vaccine efficacy" has been questioned scientifically due to contradicting evidence however, the mainstream press and journals of the professional press tend to publish more on fake news about global warming rather than the anti-immunologists who have been branded heretic.

Adults have the right to reject vaccinations, however for healthcare workers, those rights are subject to a legal battle. The new laws being considered are to require vaccinations for children health workers as well as teachers. Children in school, the option of opting out of a religious or personal convictions of parents can be "conditionally granted" by some states.

In 1905 as well as 1922, the Supreme Court rulings that are the basis of mandatory vaccinations for smallpox were both issued in outbreaks when "imminent harm" was shown due to a disease that "imperiled an entire population." The justices relied on the necessity of vaccination on having to be there that it be applied equally to all while avoiding harm to the unintentional. Mandates that are unreasonable and arbitrary could cause courts to take action. This is the case by the government mandated vaccinations given to children in school.

Parents who opt to not be vaccinated are ahead the pack in terms of public awareness about the dangers of vaccination. They are aware and not certain that the benefits of vaccination can be worth the long-term well-being. A majority of Americans who were surveyed with Pew Research Center didn't prefer mandatory shots for their children.

The survey found that 86 percent of scientists believed that during the time that members from the American Association for the Advancement of Science were asked their views on diverse "science" issues, along with a portion of people. More scientists also believed that it's safe to consume genes modified by genetic engineering, in contrast the 37% who believed general population. Do you have faith in the scientific confidence will be there in the future of vaccines derived from genetically modified genes that are now mandatory?

Scientists aren't able to prove their faith on GMO's based on proof. There were no safety tests conducted on GMO crop varieties because the vice-president Dan Quayle decreed they were similar to conventionally-bred plants. But, they believe that their "views are more in line with a completely dispassionate reading of the risks versus the benefits" for fields that they are not familiar with. "The Science is Clear!" is their motto during The Fog of War.

The claims about the safety of vaccines rest on incorrect information. The CDC found that 10% of vaccine-related injuries had been reported by physicians for the Vaccine Adverse Event Reporting System (VAERS) in 1993. There are no effective ways to boost voluntary reports by doctors were taken since then in order to guarantee safer vaccines.

The safety tests conducted for vaccines by the firms that manufacture the vaccines compare the risks to other vaccines but not placebo. To safeguard vaccine producers the parents of injured children have to be kept behind closed-doors within the Vaccine Injury Compensation Fund (VICF). These secret hearings feature a specific masters ' rulings that are not appealable. Pharmaceutical companies received immunity from damage in 1986, after civil litigation threatened their profit.

"Parents who have experienced the grueling, bureaucratic process to prove their cases say the program needs more scrutiny as California and other states tighten their vaccine laws." Tracy Siegel of the Bay Area News Group published a report in August 2015 following California Senate Bill 277, which bans medical exemptions from schoolchildren was approved. The first mention of VICF in numerous vaccine-related "news" articles in SF Bay Area media. It could also be across the state during the time of a smear campaign before Senate Bill 277 was approved.

The odds of suffering an injury are "infinitesimal, according to the CDC" however, the fund has paid $3.2 billion to more than 4,150 victims in the years since it was established. It's only the limit of a quarter million dollars in case of death, pain or suffering, yet the vast majority of settlements amount to far lower. Amy Mitten-Smith was awarded just 55,000 dollars for the brain damage her son sustained from the vaccination. She was close to missing the three-year deadline for filing for reimbursements because she'd no knowledge about the fund. She was not informed by her pediatric physician. been notified "after asking for medical attention for the [son's] reaction" in response to the vaccination.

Many parents are unaware about vaccine-related risks and report alternatives before exposing their children to vaccinations that are mandatory without their knowledge of the risks and they are not informed by their doctors following the adverse reaction. Brain damage and development delays for infants may not be detected prior to time frames imposed to parents and the victims. In spite of these hurdles to compensation, over 16,000 claims were made since 1987. 10,000 of them were dismissed without appeal. In 2005, the vast majority of the claimants are adults that were injured due to the flu vaccine.

"It's no slam dunk" Michael Firestone, a vaccine injury lawyer, was interviewed. "Cases are difficult to prove." The lawyers for the vaccine fund even are part of a national organization comprising 70 professionals. Their president has said, "We are very supportive of vaccinations, and certainly we think they are a critical aspect to health care in the U.S." Also, there is an additional legal system which pays for bills for hours.

It is funded through 75 cents tax per every vaccination. As it was only able to pay only one million doses between 2006 and 2014 According to the CDC It is in the cash. The money was never used for a public outreach campaign over the course of thirty years as an "court" of first and the last choice. In the Government Accountability Office report on the program's "long standing lack of publicity" the program is "underway".

The Center for Disease Control's (CDC) mission declaration "to promote the health and quality of life by preventing and controlling disease, injury and disability" is punctured by needles to administer vaccines. Dr. Stratton from the Institute of Medicine (IoM) declared, "the line we will not cross is to pull the vaccine, change the schedule, stop the program."

Parents and children who sacrifice for herd immunity have never been celebrated or honoured as martyrs, but vaccinations are widely praised. The lead sentence of Siegel's late report of the VICF is "Vaccines remain one of the greatest success stories in public health" with no reference to any source other than the hearsay.

QUARANTINE: THE RULE OF TYRANTS

Health officials from three California counties required that children who are healthy and unvaccinated be removed from school in the Measles Mania outbreak of 2015. The orders, which were dictatorship-like, came out without discussion or proof of how this discriminatory policy could have prevented a health crisis. The absolute authority of a designated official stems to the typhoid, smallpox and cholera outbreaks in the 19th century. both scarlet fever and measles were the most common fatalities.

Public Health Officers from Marin, Alameda and Orange counties of California prevented children who were not vaccinated not to attend school for 21 days when measles cases were detected in the schools of their children following the Disney outbreak. Measles was not a problem identified in

Marin County when Dr. Mathew Willis, PHO preemptively dictated this instruction to the county schools on January 27, 2015.

He acknowledged his belief that "it would be harmful to prevent children who are unvaccinated from attending school for the duration" however, he stated the fact that "we tend to see much more rapid spread of a disease in the event of an outbreak for communities with lower vaccination rates." The author didn't say that this as a mere remark by the CDC as well as public health officials associations without any evidence to back it up.

He was less fervent in the past year, but the doctor said "People in Marin exercise a lot of agency over their own health decisions which by and large is really a good thing." (Calling the Shots in Marin Magazine, September. 2014)

Two cases of measles within Marin students were discovered on the same day the next day, Dr. Willis's decision was questioned. "These [siblings] were out of school before and throughout any infectious period, they have been safely isolated from the community and will remain isolated for the next three weeks" Therefore, the decision to exclude students who had not been vaccinated was not enforced. He didn't want to defend a arbitrary restriction of vaccination.

One child was afflicted with measles, in 2016, at an Nevada County, CA charter school, the whole school was shut for just one day. Then the children that were not following vaccination schedules were barred from attending for a total of two weeks. The majority of kindergarteners within the school's area aren't fully protected. The issue was discovered two weeks after the last time the child was at school. The symptoms generally show up a week later but a wait of three weeks could be possible but not likely. (SF Chronicle, 3/30/16)

The majority of schools are funded by the state that are based on attendance. So being unable to send dozens of kids away for a period of three weeks, whether excused or not, will be bound to result in negative consequences. There was no need for research to be conducted by Willis to end students' quarantine, and not to speak the possibility of economic harm for attendance-based schools or parents who work. The chance that the students could self- quarantine at home is not high and any protection offered by schools is lost in the mall.

According to CDC The CDC estimates that the CDC estimates that 22 million days of school are lost due to common cold every year. This is despite no vaccination and 38 million affected by flu-like illnesses that are grouped together as influenza-related viruses. The CDC wants schools to "encourage students and staff to get annual influenza vaccinations." But there is still no quarantine in place for children who haven't received the flu vaccine they were required.

There is no evidence that the Measles, Mumps and Rubella (MMR) or measles rubella Measles Rubella (MR) vaccines have the same effectiveness as they claim in the prevention of measles. The editor-in-chief of the prestigious journal Vaccine asked "the public health establishment to accept that the measles vaccine is unworkable" in an article that was published in an Canadian financial publication in the year 2012. The doctor. Gregory Poland consults with the CDC as well as Merck, the Defense Department and Merck and is the director of Mayo Clinic's vaccine studies and developments. He is planning to promote the latest, more effective measles vaccine. He had been promoting it as a potential investment. He also noted that Dr. Poland noted the "paradoxical situation whereby measles in highly immunized societies occurs primarily among those previously immunized." His opinions weren't widely discussed in the south.

Twenty-one students were diagnosed measles in a class "with a documented immunization level of 100%" during the early 1980's. The CDC announced a recently reported measles outbreaks in regions that have 98% vaccination rate. Measles outbreaks are increasing within highly immunized nations like China that have 99% vaccination rates in 2013, according to World Health Organization data. What's the beefy herd immune system?

The majority of measles patients were given two doses of measles vaccination during an measles outbreak that occurred in Canada. The outbreak began when a vaccinated educator contracted measles while on holiday. Unknown percentages of measles cases that occur in those who have been twice vaccinated aren't recognized since it is because they "were immunized." No person can tell who is likely to be ill after exposure to the disease, no matter if they are vaccine-vaccinated or not. Therefore, randomly assigned unvaccinated and vaccinated youngsters should be placed in screening to ensure fairness.

Students miss school due to sickness, but the majority of them don't die. There aren't vaccines to fight illnesses that cause coughs, colds stomach bugs, colds or "flu-like illnesses" causing most absences. Days lost from the 8% of students in school children,(10 percentage of boys) with a history of illness however suffer from ADHD and learning difficulties due to vaccination-related injuries have not been estimated. The causality hasn't been investigated yet, even though the damage caused by biological components of vaccines is known.

It is believed that the MMR vaccine (the single measles vaccination was withdrawn) makes use of live virus. The virus is weakened or attenuated and measles-inducing instances are recorded. "Measles

Mary" was written about in a study published in 2012 published in Clinical Infectious Disease. Mary became sick following vaccination, and then infected other people with the virus strain that is vaccine-resistant which was half of the population who were vaccinated. If schoolchildren who are exempt from vaccination or adults who have a weak immune system hurry to receive vaccinations, they'll be among the likely carriers of the subsequent virus outbreak.

Dr. Willis from Marin said that two doses of the MMR have 99% effectiveness against measles. The CDC says 97% and the doctor from. Poland estimated only 90 percent. Everyone acknowledges that the effectiveness of vaccines decreases over time. The need for booster shots is assessed in blood samples that are tested for titers in serum of viral counts, much like oil alters. "Poor responders" who produced lower levels of antibodies following an MMR injection did not remain protected even after more shots and had a six-fold higher risk of becoming susceptible to contracting measles in outbreaks over "high responders", Dr. Poland found. Children and adults with a decline in vaccinations are also exempt from all schools that have measles cases, as well as those who are not responding and should be exempted in order to maintain impartiality. Anyone who has had measles get lifetime immunity.

If "epidemics" of these childhood disease are seen among those who have been vaccine-vaccinated, the information is hidden in footnotes, patients who are not diagnosed and obscurant data. Measles can be misdiagnosed due to the fact that there are many other infections that trigger flares, rashes and fevers. It was found that the British Public Health Laboratory found an 97.5 percentage error rate when they examined the saliva of 2,000 kids whose physicians were able to diagnose measles.

Measles diagnosed by a lab that are the same type as the vaccine are acceptable in quarantine based on scientific evidence. The vaccine would not have been able to be used in those Disney Measles cases, since they had an Asian variant and not by the American virus strain that is found within the MMR.

The death of a patient and the disabling injury are rare due to measles, and this is true even in the Third World countries where patients receive vitamin A and D, or the cod liver oil. The measles mortality rate in America is almost zero. There were 12 hospital visits, but no deaths California for the duration of four months of measles. Disney measles "epidemic".

Health crises that are happening in the modern world are not considered by the Totalitarian Inoculationists. Over the course of four months the measles mania, 66,000 asthma sufferers were treated in California hospitals, 10,000 of them were admitted to hospitals and 120 perished according to annual rates of cases with asthma. The most vulnerable include African American and poor children less than five. MediCal covers the majority of the billion-dollar cost of treatment, and yearly payouts that amount to $750million. Diesel-powered buses, diesel vehicles and wood-burning fires emit asthma triggers. Do you think you or the Public Health Officer quarantine them?

Guns kill up to 80 pre-school kids each year. twenty children and teenagers get shot every day across the U.S. Homicides involving guns are a common occurrence on the social media networks on the internet as a study from 2018 Chicago study discovered.

Six million children aged 5-14 years old get taken to emergency rooms due to accident-related injuries every year. An additional 8 million 15-24 year olds receive ER being treated after traffic accidents or falls, sports, poisoning, and fires as well as others "accidents". Children die more often due to being hit by driveways, or left in hot automobiles than from any of illnesses that have been vaccinated across the U.S., including lab confirmed influenza (not the exaggerated numbers that the CDC boasts about, but mostly due to pneumonia.)

The most frequent reason for deaths among youngsters and teens and can kill up to 10,000 every year. Ralph Nader's fight for automobile security pushed safer vehicles from Detroit and Washington and Mothers Against Drunk Drivers forced the strictest DUI regulations and enforcement. The group reduced the number of deaths from traffic by about 20,000 annually from 1970's high, but the top spot for fatalities remains the same.

Chapter 3: The Selling Of Sb 277

The effort to end parents' choice to subject their children to compulsory vaccination in order to attend the school in California was launched in the year 2010. Pertussis Panic led to mandatory booster shots for seventh graders. Parents who decided to not give their child the shot due to personal reasons must first talk to a physician and inform parents about the "facts".

The plant was fertilized by the Dr. Paul Offit's novel Do You Believe in Magic? The Sense and Nonsense of Alternative Medicine. Jerome Groopman, the "quackbuster" who reviewed the book favorably the in The New Republic October, 2013, did not mention the fact that Proffit. "Proffit"' patented an rotavirus vaccination where numerous babies suffered injuries and died shortly after the injection. Proffit claims that Dr. Proffit claims there was just an "temporal association."

Eula Biss's lengthy article Sentimental Medicine: Why We Still Aren't Thrilled by Vaccines(Harper's Magazine , January. 2013) was a precursor to On Immunity, her highly praised book about vaccines that was published in 2014. The book is not viewed as highly in the chapter 17 of this book.

Call for Parents to Get Vaccinated called for the public shame of parents who refused to let their children benefit from compulsory vaccinations. (San Francisco Chronicle Op-Ed, 9/9/14) Steve Heilig, the creator of the article, said that "the primary factor" for exclusions is "fears about risks of vaccines-especially of autism." The author claimed that this was due to "conspiracy theories and mistrust" and linked them to the deaths of vaccine makers "in some nations." The author was referring to Pakistan however any responsibility for conspiracy theories or distrust of vaccines within the Muslim world is attributed to the false vaccination programme which was employed to find and kill Osama Bin Osama Bin Laden.

USA Today published a similar editorial that called for a halt to the religious exemption for vaccinations within the U.S. (4/13/2014), nevertheless, they gave Barbara Loe Fisher of the National Vaccine Information Center space to speak out. The Vaccine Information Center's director turned the tables saying "non-medical exemptions to vaccination protect people as well as the entire community from dangerous effective vaccines and oppression. If the State is able to force individuals against their wishes to receive biological substances with unknown toxicities today it will not be able to put a limitation on freedoms that individuals which the State is able to remove to serve bettering the world tomorrow." National newspaper's readers' polls overwhelmingly favored vaccine exemptions based on philosophical, religious or religious beliefs.

Marin Magazine climbed on this rapid-growing pro-vaxx social media trend by launching a campaign called Calling the Shotsin September 2014. It seemed to be a little more balanced and contained the words of the Marin pediatrician who notably delayed and dispersed the recommended vaccination schedule for infants as well as toddlers as well as a mom who refused to give her child vaccines from vaccinations due to unknown issues.

Rebuttals from local public health officials reaffirmed the prevailing view that vaccinations aren't a cause of autism, and the epidemic of diseases that have been eradicated could recur because of the exemptors in a small percentage. The report didn't dispute this assertion with evidence to prove them wrong, but a trend of medical transcription was repeatedly that was repeated repeatedly in the subsequent months.

There was Ebola In the course of that campaign season. It proved that Americans were able to be brought into fear and panic due to disease, particularly those from that "Dark Continent." The Disney Measles Mania was seized by the media to increase fear the following winter. The Los Angeles Times editorial blamed exemptions' "anti-science stubbornness" in early January 2015 for creating the recurrence in "a disease that has been beaten by modern medicine." Outbreak puts the spotlight on the anti-vaccine movement(Associated Press, 1/23/15) revealed a couple of dozen measles cases as if Contagion was likely. "As one of the world's biggest tourist destinations, Disney was a perfect spot for the virus to spread, with large numbers of babies too young to be vaccinated and lots of visitors from countries that do not require measles shots." In contrast to this LA Times conclusion of cause.

CrazyClusters (SF Chronicle editorial from 1/25/15) described the findings of a Kaiser Permanente study showing geographic the high number of under-vaccinated and non-vaccinated children living in "well educated, affluent" regions. The study slammed parents because they were "refusing to give your children the proper number of vaccinations [,which] shows a lack of courage and taking responsibility." Kaiser researchers concluded that the groups "deserved focused intervention." The Chronicle ominously warned, "The state may need to step in and take more serious steps to avoid threats to the public health."

The editorial cartoon that appeared in the issue also showed measles virus-infected Disney Dwarf Doc facing his infectious agents, as well as a woman who was wearing a Moms against Vaccines shirt as well as her children eating ice cream. Mickey is taken into the Small World Quarantine Center in the background.

Over 1,000 In Arizona Are Watched For Measles-7 Confirmed Cases Ahead of Super Bowl. (New York Times, January 30, 2015) stated that health officials had an out-of-control panic across California's state neighbor. Will Humble, the Arizona health director, demanded "residents who have not been vaccinated and who might have been exposed to stay home from school, work or day care for 21 days." Dr. Cara Christ, the State's chief medical officer, acknowledged the 4.7 percentage of exemptions for AZ. "It allows the disease to get into those areas and establish a foothold, and once it establishes a foothold, it's very, very difficult to control." For these Chicken Little officials, measles outbreaks dwindled quickly, after the outbreak was declared to be over at the end of April. But, it was enough to contaminate the water of perception.

The mania grew and spread, I reprinted numerous articles, editorial cartoons, and letters that were published in local newspapers as well as south Florida newspapers on a one-week stay in February. It was not fair or well-balanced report on this Disney Measles outbreak and SB277 legislation within The SF Bay Area daily and weekly papers I perused. Also, neither was Florida looking for research. The fact that vaccines are NoBrainer(The Florida Keys Keynoter, 2/18/15) is not talking about the brain damage caused by vaccines. It hit the pulpit "in our mind, willfully exposing one's child to a contagious disease borders on abuse."

The campaign was made clear to be an international campaign when Congress introduced the Vaccines Save Lives Resolution, declaring that "no credible evidence" proves that vaccines cause "life threatening or disabling disease" in spite of having established the Vaccine Injury Compensation Fund thirty years earlier to compensate the parents of children who were who were injured or killed by vaccines. Four supporters had gotten more than $200k in contributions to their campaigns in 2014.

Twelve states have had proposed laws that would have banned exemptions from the right of Freedom of Choice in Health Care to their child through the elimination of any personal, philosophical or religious exclusions. Medical exemptions are the only exception. California was the goal they had their eye on. The state was taken in massive mediasteria and shaken the state until lawmakers gave up.

The Marin Independent Journal got on the bandwagon by releasing a front-page report; Outbreak puts focus on vaccine options. (Marin IJ 2/1/15) The full-color photo of six-year-old Rhett Krawitt was highlighted. The photo showed him holding soda cans held in his palms, possibly completely natural. The treatment for leukemia left him with a compromised immune system to withstand vaccines. His father was angry, as "he couldn't count on others for protection" in the context to"the "social compact." If there was a chance that he would contract the doctor told him, "It might delay his cancer treatment." The kid became a favored face of the news media while his dad dragged his son around public hearings despite the medical advice to stay away from crowds and enclosed places. He was the unofficial advocate of CA laws that banned exempting school children from vaccinations with the exception of those similar to those who are at risk of being harmed by vaccines or even kill. Parents would be hesitant to grant exemption in the event they could be aware of the risks that their child could suffer.

The day senator Dick Pan of Sacramento proposed Senate Bill 277 to the California Senate on February 4, 2015 the media's almost constant campaign against exemptors started. The same day, U.S.

Senators Barbara Boxer and Diane Feinstein wrote to the state's top health officer, saying "We believe there should be no such thing as a philosophical or personal belief exemption, since everyone uses public spaces."

Science and public health must prevail,(SF Chronicle editorial 2/4/15) The editorial strongly warned that "In a decent society, public health and safety trump myths not based on science." The Vaccine Avoiders pose a threat to the state (SF Chronicle 2/8/15) Included a graphic that compared California's relaxed vaccination rules against the rest of the world. 20 other states offered the similar exemptions to California. Other states allowed religious exemptions, with the exception of Mississippi as well as West Virginia. There was no irony in the fact that California's law would correct our unforgiving laws, taking a step in the path of public health laws in states that have the most severe childhood health outcomes compared to Arkansas.

The graph that accompanies it of the rates of exemption for kindergarteners showed that rates rose slightly following a 1998 British study that linked vaccinations to autism. The rate increased by three times in the wake of numerous studies conducted by government agencies as well as news articles "proving vaccines do not cause autism" have been published at the beginning of the millennium. It is below 3% in the entire state and is well over the 90percent needed for the conferring of herd immunity. The Hearst controlled Chronicle was reportedly intent on launching another war of yellow journalism with this one focusing on parental rights.

The columnist for their weekly edition, Joe Mathews proposed publicizing the names of parents that excluded their children from school like sexual offenders. (2/15/2015) The continued silence will "deny me the power to make a decision about whether my children ought to be in the houses of parents who have shrewdly chosen to stay to stay away from the modern world. The harassment of any kind must be avoided" He tolerantly said. Alvin Gross of San Francisco believes that unvaccinated children ought to become "identifiable by wearing a button or ribbon to protect other children from making contact" while avoiding the nazi identification system. (SF Chronicle, 4/17/ 2015)

Many letters and articles to the editor have been poured over the parents with many questioning the prevalent trend. The comedian John Stewart jumped into the controversy, accusing Marin parents to be "science denying, affluent California liberals practicing mindful stupidity" and rim shot. Jimmy Kimmel mocked Marin parents for being "more frightened of gluten than smallpox." Time magazine columnist Joe Klein condemned the "crazy, nutso talk about vaccines" and called to have "moderation- a grown up and civil" public discussion about political issues. (3/9/15) National Geographic's March cover the month of The War on Science, mixing vaccine fear with the moon landing and global warming hoaxers.

The presidential candidate was a clogging Republican presidential scrums entered the discussion. Three of them were criticized in the press for their support of the rights of parents to exclude from their children. New Jersey. Governor Chris Christie, Kentucky Senator Rand Paul and billionaire Donald Trump initially backed Freedom of Choice. Christie quickly retracted his support for the "measure of choice" for parents. He displayed a surprising amount of pace for such a large man.

Sen. Paul is a medical doctor but was put in with the anti-science garbage in the bin. Paul has since denied that vaccinations can cause problems, after declaring that he "heard of many children who wound up with profound mental disorders after vaccinations." Paul could have mentioned his father, Texas Congressman Ron Paul, "If fear of infection caused by unvaccinated people justifies the need for mandatory vaccination laws, then why don't officers be able to fine or even arrest individuals who aren't covering their mouths or noses when they cough or wheeze while in public?"The liberal section of the party has been snubbed in the discussion.

Trump continued to be uncompromising, possibly helping him to be at the highest results in polls.

Hilary Clinton tweeted "the science is conclusive. The Earth is round The sky is blue, and the vaccines do the job." However, she was not as confident during the 2008 presidential election, where she and presidential candidate Barak Obama "left to the chance that there was a connection between vaccinations as well as autism. Both said that the need for more research was urgent." Both condemned the "anti-scientific" debate in the year 2015. Clinton's witty tweet was not a good idea in her polls.

Jim Carey tweeted and Robert F. Kennedy, Jr. traveled to California to protest against this legislation in February. Kennedy addressed his home at the Commonwealth Club in San Francisco and at a large public gathering in Sacramento. News reports of his speech did not report on his ferocious condemnation of CDC as the "cesspool of corruption, including scandalous conflicts with the $25 billion vaccine industry." It was not reported that "hundreds of peer-reviewed studies have shown that Thimerosal as a mercury-containing preservative, is a debilitating poison linked to neurological diseases which are currently affecting American children."Thimerosal"Let the Science Talk by Kennedy, a book co-written with two medical professionals, references these studies, as well as notes "39 studies strongly suggesting that Thimerosal causes autism." However, Kennedy continues to be branded "a proponent of the discredited theory that vaccines cause autism." After he started working alongside Donald Trump after his election to examine the harms of vaccination, his group, the San Francisco Robert F. Kennedy Democratic Club, "started to get hate mail about being associated with a prominent anti vaxxer." (SF Chronicle, 22nd February 2017)

The Dr. Andrew Wakefield was "covered" by The Chronicle for his stance against the law during a lecture at Life Chiropractic College in Hayward, CA. Dr. Andrew Wakefield was still known by the Chronicle as "the discredited doctor" because his 1998 research paper linking MMR vaccine to autism was pulled by Lancet but in 2014, the British High Court quashed all accusations against doctors who wrote the paper along with the doctor.

The news was never reported in the dozens of reports in the corporate media about his journey from prophetic to heretic. The late Dr. Wakefield was unrepentant, "It does not matter if die in my grave discredited. There is nothing I can lose today. It's a crucial matter. Parents no longer have to have the responsibility of their children."

He didn't get the study he conducted in 2009 in NeuroToxicology which showed a delay in the development of the newborn monkeys that receive Hepatitis B vaccination. The vaccine is also routinely offered to new American newborns. Premature or overweight monkeys are at greatest the risk.

Doctor. Art Reingold, a UC Berkeley epidemiologist who helped develop national policies on childhood vaccination got the final say. "At the moment, he's going all the time as a hero for the people who oppose vaccination. When something gets stuck within people's heads, the research that follows could not offer them enough evidence. There is a possibility of a lasting impact that can create harm for the public." Reingold has ignored the growing evidence from both legal and scientific sources of his vaccine policies leading to a health crisis for the public because of this prejudice.

Editors' letters almost always accused parents who are exempt from parental responsibility of returning measles, smallpox, polio, pertussis or even the disease. They rebuked them for bad parental behavior, social responsibility and challenged their sanity. They compared them to fake global warming skeptics and Earth-centered solar system apologists, claiming on their "critical thinking, thorough investigations and weighing of the evidence." Many were unsure of the reason the best educated parents are "anti-science", or mentioned some reasonable concerns regarding medical procedures, proving to be the 3rd leading cause of death for Americans.

Many editorials and letters call for passage of SB 277. Parents who not been in the spotlight prior to this bill, from the possibility that they would be "being vilified and ostracized" as well as other similar-minded individuals including vegan mothers to Black Muslims. A large number of people protested the bill at the Golden Gate Bridge, in Sacramento as well as at various public hearings. Peaceful assemblies in Sacramento were granted the media attention, however very little information was leaked through the media or on airwaves.

Carl Krawitt continued bringing his son Rhett to public hearings, in spite of health warnings from doctors that immune compromised people "should avoid crowds if possible." Wear the respirator mask in case they do this. It would have made him sound a bit sluggish but. The fears of exempted children that could be infected by his son were extensively discussed, however government guidelines advising against having close contact with "recently vaccinated" people were ignored. The spread of measles pertussis, chicken pox and rotavirus as well as influenza smallpox and polio viruses by people who were recently vaccinated is well confirmed, with those who are immune compromised being the highest risk.

The legislation was approved by the Senate Health Committee on April 10, despite the fervent pleas of parents. Karen Kain, whose daughter died from mercury-preserved vaccine, questioned "Who is allowed the decision today of which babies matter more? Since the risk is there and there is a choice, it must be made." (SF Chronicle 2/10/15)

RFK, Jr. spoke of his rally again in Sacramento just prior to the vote warning "the checks and balances of the democratic system which are meant to be a barrier between corporate power and our kids have been taken away. There's just one obstacle left, and that's our parents. " He helped to kill similar legislation in Oregon as well as Washington in the months prior to this. In California He was in the news on the basis of his linking vaccination-related deaths and injuries in"the "holocaust" , not his proof of the mercury-rich shots that poison children. He upset those who put this mass slaughter in the same category as"the High Holies.

Doctor. Dean Blumberg, a pediatrician, who testified on behalf of both the American Academy of Pediatrics and the California Medical Society, delivered the traditional dogma "Let me clarify. There is no controversy in science concerning the effectiveness and safety of vaccinations. There is no room for disagreement between mainstream doctors as well as scientists." The law was supported by groups representing hospital doctors, physicians as well as teachers, public healthcare officials, the local government schools boards, unions and doctors as well as a "silent majority" of parents.

A vocal minority that opposed it, "generated more phone calls than any other measure this year" to lawmakers. Many of them included the threat of death and curses from religious groups. Sen. Pan and the bill's co-sponsor enlisted armed guards for a short period. The bill was blocked by the Senate Education Committee the next week, on April 16 because of "facing a barrage of questions [Sen. Pan] could not answer about the right of California children to attend public schools, even if they are unvaccinated."

The delay was met with severe editorials and stories praising inept politicians. among them, Vaccination Bill BucklesUnder

Parent's Pressureheadlined in a Chronicle report. Senator. Pan doubled down by draggin the "iron lung" out of the basement of a hospital with old people who were crippled by the polio virus (or in the case of Cutter Lab produced Salk vaccine and causing what was described as the "largest polio epidemic in American history.") The vaccine went through several Senate Committees and then the whole Senate with just four votes leave in May's final days.

The bill eliminated requirements that parents are informed about the vaccination rates at their schools and also granted the new "medical exemptions" for students who already have an exemption. The bill allowed for conditional admission to students in kindergarten who resisted certain mandatory vaccines. The bill also permitted exempted children to have their children home-schooled as independent study groups. It also made sure special education students get all the services they require from their schools when they meet the requirements to be eligible for Individualized Education Programs and most important, it allowed grandfathered-in exemptions for children who are already enrolled in order to divide the conflict.

Children's parents have been the most targeted. They'll have fight to the end in consultation with their physicians and their representatives, or suffer the consequences of those "unavoidable" harms of vaccination. An analysis of pediatricians revealed that more parents delayed vaccines or delaying them of those on the CDC schedule. Parents were most concerned about the long-term effects of the five or more shots they receive during the course of a visit to a physician against 14 diseases at the age of two and beginning with Hepatitis B that is which is a sexually transmitted illness. They were skeptical of the pharmaceutical industry along with the medical and government establishments that were found to collaborate with them in creating numerous health disasters. The majority of pediatricians agreed to the delay, in spite of public warnings that avoiding the vaccination "puts kids at risk for getting vaccine preventable diseases and might lead to disease outbreaks."

"A savvy public with ever greater levels of medical knowledge is growing frustrated with the absolute pronouncements of modern medicine and will likely challenge them" Medical doctors from Toronto University Health Network wrote of parents who "spent hundreds of hours reviewing medical studies, books and news stories and networking on social media." The reality is that many doctors would rather challenge a parent who has more knowledge about vaccinations than the bare minimum of CDC speaking points. Medical schools have the least amount of time to educate themselves about vaccines as opposed to nutrition education, which is essentially the only thing they study. They prefer to remain in disbelief from their willful ignorance since their work is contingent on the administration of these poisons without any question. Pediatricians in some states have banned the exclusion of parents from the practice. However, other doctors are more discreetly welcoming their patients.

The CA Assembly passed their amended bill on June 25. Two Republicans were in favor, and just five Democrats did not support the bill. They also allowed religious or personal exemptions to new vaccines that were that were added to the mandatory schedules. They also broadened the reach of doctors when they provide medical exemptions in the context of family history and negative reactions to vaccines. The loophole can be wide enough that it covers those who have the basis of their religious or personal convictions, therefore any gain gained in the number of vaccinations will be wiped out if doctors accurately ask about the history of family members with immune-mediated disorders.

The Senate approved the bill as amended on June 29 before delivering it to Gov. Jerry Brown. The opposition filed a petition that had more than 50,000 signatures, asking Governor. Brown to reject the proposal and supporters gathered 37,000 signatures. There was speculation on what direction Brown could go. "The three great mysteries in life are the Holy Trinity, transubstantiation and Jerry Brown's mind," declared Jack Pitney, a McKenna College political scientist instructor.

The Catholic Church did not take a position on the issue despite it being pro-life. Science has proven that vaccines are the leading reason for the death of neonates and infants. There is no opposition to the fallout from nuclear power plants, pesticides or other commercial chemicals that cause death to fetuses Only surgical abortions are available for women who opt to have them.

Kristen Hundley, president of Our Children, Our Choice was "hopeful that Governor Brown is a defender of his commitment to the First Amendment to the U.S. Constitution. We are aware that Governor Brown is an advocate of precision medicine. This is directly in opposition to the notion of medical mandates that do not allow for a one-size-fits every approach."

However, this isn't the governor "Moonbeam" Brown of the 1970's. The governor of today is "corporate fascist" Jerry Brown like Jim Carey tweeted. It's true that Jerry Brown was the former state attorney general who convicted a handful of corporations in the state that has no shortage of. The Brown is the patron of billionaires and a the global warming critic, and pro-fracking governor. The final result is that the governor's Jesuit and Zen brain didn't think long before he signed the bill into law on the final day of June, 2015.

"The scientific evidence is conclusive that vaccinations greatly shield children from the risk of dangerous and infectious disease. It is clear that immunization effectively protects and benefits the entire community." Brown wrote in his declaration of signature with no reference to any.

Sen. Pan was less measured in his triumphant crowing "The scientific evidence is conclusive. It is now impossible to spread infectious disease or outbreaks. not more hospitalizations, there are no more deaths, and no fears." Ding-dong The Witch is dead! The battle soon became more personal when residents in his Sacramento district started circulating the petition for his recall. The district had until December.

Chapter 4: California Parents Survival Strategy

I wouldn't ever advise parents to not vaccinate their kids*. But those who advocate vaccination insist that we immunize our children to be able to go to "all California schools and child care facilities, including child care centers, day nurseries, nursery schools, family day care homes and development centers, whether public or private" as required by the law.

Exiting the state might be an unsustainable choice since it is a campaign that's conducted at the state level. It is better to take on an action of rearguard within the Golden State and make them be wary of extending their reach in other states. The best strategy is to develop a method which creates alliances to removal using a variety of strategies employing legal strategies already in use.

An action that challenges the constitutionality of Senate Bill 277 might have more chances of being invalidated than petitions for voter approval. A law that strips parents of their right to reject potentially deadly medicines for their child is the immediate protection of the public as well as a procedure that has been proven to work and isn't more harmful than the advantages derived from the initial Supreme Court decision on mandatory vaccinations. The proponents of this legislation will have a hard time proving their exaggerated, unsubstantiated claims by proving their legality, but they aren't required to.

The Head On lawsuits have been fighting to enter the courtroom, let alone get the upper hand. The motion of the state to dismiss the lawsuit that was filed against the California's SB277 was approved by an federal court on 13 January 17. "Unlike the previous lawsuits the lawsuit is focused on the constitutional rights. It is worth noting that the United States Supreme Court has consistently affirmed that Americans have a right to bodily autonomy. This is the right to deny unwelcome medical procedures. The Court has repeatedly ruled that parents are entitled to a fundamental right to control the education for their child. Additionally, the California Supreme Court has held that public education for children is an inherent right of the State of California. The interplay between rights forms the basis of our lawsuit. Our argument is based on the most cherished principles. The government is not able to force you into giving the exercise of one right in exchange for you would like to exercise a different one" the founder of Voice for Choice Christina Hildebrand said.

"The federal judge essentially punted. The judge stated that since the right of education is a constitutional state right, she was going to give the state courts a sway in enforcing the right. We think this is a strange outcome, because the constitutional rights of state citizens to education is obviously interwoven here with rights of parental autonomy and medical autonomy under the federal law and parental-discretion rights, we think the ruling is in our favor, and we believe that we'll be eventually rewarded. The federal district court is joined by with other district courts of the federal government in concluding that excessively burdensome vaccine regulations violate the right to public education that, while not recognized by the federal government but is recognized by California."

The establishment of education allows the medical/legal collusion to mandate mandatory vaccinations for their students without questioning the justification or the proof. The students are either uninformed or unsupported when they challenge the basis of this interference on the mission of their institution. The bill is set to put in the future legal procedures that may render the entire system illegal or unconstitutional. Blind faith in the supremacy of law that provides justice is the same as blind faith in vaccines that offer healthcare. Even with constitutional safeguards against the power of a state religious institution, medical orthodoxy can sentence children to irreparable harm or even death, without any due process or public testimony.

There are fewer direct paths toward the end purpose in repeal, other than lawsuits or citizens' ballot initiatives. If you are a California parent decides to not vaccine their child, despite constant propaganda, the majority of public opinion, or legal obstacles There are exceptions to the no-exemption law. Utilizing the exemptions included in the bill could create into a rift between those who aren't influenced by many of our citizens who aren't well-informed.

In order to pass SB277, it was necessary to make several amendments in order to please the Democrat majority who supported the bill. Republicans were merely stomping and puffed in the background about defending personal liberties, or about the fact that religious and private schools were also included instead of defending the dismissal of a constitutional obligation of the state to ensure the same access to public schools. The only difference was that neither Democrat or Republican (there there weren't any non-partisans) representatives mentioned the plethora of data proving massive negative effects versus insignificant benefits, due to being equally ignorant as the majority of their fellow citizens or were not capable of navigating the haze of conflict with concise sounds. The tongue-tied argument is the issue MV=TI aims to resolve.

What do parents do? A new modification "grandfathered" in children already who were enrolled in schools. Parents using religion-based or philosophical exclusions for their students prior to the 1st of January, 2016 did not lose those rights in the event that they continued to reside in the district they that they were registered with. If they moved or transferred to a different district, the laws that states "no shots-no school" kicked into effect (still subject to legal challenge regardless of whether the law specifically states this). The rights were revoked for children who were in kindergarten or pre-school for the school year 2016/2017.

This split the opposition of parents which was already small and unorganized as older children were not at risk so long as they didn't move schools. Parents with young children tend to be overwhelmed. they only start to become anti-vaxxers when their child's injuries are which is even more than they are. But parents who slid across the finish line before closing of the locks should be supportive to the ones who were left behind. This book, as well as this method is mine.

A second amendment disqualified children from qualifying to receive the Individualized Education Plan, (IEP) because of physical, mental and learning or behavioral disabilities due to federal law that protect the rights of such youngsters to equal accessibility to education. Most often, the disabilities are caused by vaccinations, but symptoms may be detected too long after injections for them to qualify for compensation. There is a wide range of options with 13 disabilities that are eligible to be considered for inclusion. Some of them have broad diagnostic options with a wide range of specialists. Schools are obliged to conduct tests to determine if a person has a disabilities upon request from parents and must consider Independent Educational Evaluations. They are required to pay for all education services needed by a child in order to provide equality of access as well as the child must have an Individualized Education Plan, so they are in a position of a stake in denying diagnosis.

However, there's a legal framework that gives parents a variety of rights to redress their choice, arising out schools' refusing to pay for an equal education. (The Disability Rights Education and Defense Fund) It isn't wise to try using the tools available to exclude your child's education through the IEP diagnosis. In the event that you want to convince schools to push to repeal SB277 in light of the cost increase and their administrative delay in disadvantaging diagnosis. It is possible that they will be happy with the lower costs resulting from fewer vaccine-damaged students if this became a reality, but it rarely comes to fruition.

A different school-based exemption can be granted to students who are in Independent Studies Programs not receiving education in a classroom. The majority of school districts offer or have the ability to set up such programs, if asked by parents. The program doesn't require a diagnosis this makes ISP's less of a barrier and stigmatized that IEP's. ISP's are subject to interpretation by local authorities, including what is considered a classroom however students need to have access to all the opportunities that other students have in the district. Teachers, be it online or in person (usually there is a "guide" oversees several IEP's) Participating in arts and sports activities as well as counseling, field excursions library and gathering spaces.

They are essentially open to public funding for community and home schools. Certain are run through charter schools or are co-educational home schools. This is more expensive and time-consuming for schools to offer such. If enough parents sign up their children and notify school officials that they're doing this in order to not have a mandatory vaccine This could also create an effective pressure on schools to vote in favor of removal.

Home schooling is an exemption and it requires setting up the school in your home and submitting a Private School Affadavit. These can be set up as cooperatives, where parents share duties so no parent is full time educator/administrator. (research via The Home School Association of California) Private schools may also provide satellite home programs that take care of certain paperwork and also provide oversight for education.

The routes are difficult to negotiate as compared to a medical exemption granted by an authorized physician. It is the sole exemption that is still permitted by law. There are a limited number of pediatricians ready to issue letters exempting kids from the vaccination schedule in order to allow school attendance. As a cautionary shot, the doctor. Bob Sears (author of The Vaccine Book and a FaceBook page that has thousands of followers)was one of the first people to be questioned by the California

Medical Board for doing the same thing in September. They claimed he acted without having a "complete detailed medical history." They also the board accused him of doing something "grossly negligent and depart[ing] from standard of care." Dr. Bob could lose his medical license and could become a Wakefield model.

This was just one of the 54 claims regarding exemptions to vaccinations which the CMB had received during the year. the majority of which were just cautioned. It's not clear the number of complaints involving doctors who refused to sign the an exemption letter, but it shouldn't be a bad idea to submit one even in the event that your doctor doesn't. Actually, it may make them busy enough to pursue those who are exemptor friends. In the meantime, Osteopathic Medical Board has no disciplinary action against physicians who signed exemptors at the time.

Doctor. Sears actually gave vaccinations and spread the 10 vaccines California must have for attendance at school on a larger timeframe and only gave one dose per visit. He wrote that "it is imperative that all families and doctors operate within the guidelines of the law and the standards of care" on his Facebook page prior to when the charges were brought against him. He also acknowledged letters for temporary entry as well as medical exemptions to children who he believed to be legitimately qualified for based on the immediate relatives' history of autoimmune disorders or previous serious reactions to vaccinations from the child's parents or siblings, a the current medical condition or illness of the child or siblings, the presence of autism, behavioral or learning issues within the immediate family or allergy in the child, or several members of the same family.

In recognition of his advocacy for the public and fair-minded attitude to vaccination, he was targeted and used as an example to others doctors. There aren't many physicians who be able to agree or issue profession's license on the risk factors listed above, however they will generally exclude children with compromised immune systems from treatments for cancer as well as other illnesses.

The process of converting your pediatrician into an exempting friend will likely necessitate a long-term plan since very few have performed independently and accept the public's opinion. Begin by assembling a precise and complete medical histories of your family and submitting it during regular newborn checkups. Reassure them that they are not putting off the appointment and analyzing the evidence. Refuse any arguments against the recording of these risk factors in arguing that they are well-known risks for vaccination "adverse events."

Provide documentation and provide them with the Dr. Sears balanced book with numerous citations to scientific research. Ask them to take on continuing education. Be aware that most students learnt not much about vaccinations in medical school, and more about nutrition. Coca-Cola is a significant donor for the American Academy of Pediatrics and they're not revealing the amount of vaccine makers contribute to charity.

Stop the school from being cut off further by avoiding pre-school as well as kindergarten (which generally are Petri dishes to treat common diseases and parasites with none of the vaccines or viruses released from children who have recently been vaccinated). In the first grade, you must have the requirement of a "conditional entry", which will require a physician to sign off the conditional entry once. If the school you attend insists on confirming the vaccination, (some don't care, but when you hear about it through the media, move if you can) Start your vaccinations by using the Tdap If you decide to spread these out in the manner your requirements of your school or follow the plan B, C or D.

You can ask him or her sharp questions about their vaccination practices and they will accept their ignorance and willingness to conduct an investigation or tell that you should leave and go to an alternative physician. What are they aware of about what is known as the Vaccine Adverse Events Reporting System? Do they have a history of reporting any vaccine-related injury to VAERS? Are they aware of the steps to report it? Are they aware of the batch numbers for the current supply of vaccines for the purpose of reporting should they suffer an accident? Do they have one dose vaccines to supplement typical triple combinations?

How long are they monitoring babies for signs of fever and breathing issues, or tears that are inconsolable, and seizures after injection? Should they report a problem to VAERS if parents had informed them of these typical reactions once they had left the facility? Do they want to be a witness in front of an official of the Vaccine Accident Compensation Fund should this vaccine caused serious injury or even death for my child?

It could end up being a loss, since their fear of exile and the reduction in income and fame is more than enough to be a good parent for the ignorant. Still, it's not a cost-effective use of time and energy because, as more parents challenge their theories, anti-vaxx doctors are going to realize that they cannot provide answers to basic questions about their methods and their theories. Doctors must assume the role of"the captain" of the ship and this can cause the doctors to conduct more investigation and uncover how their perception of the world was manipulated. The doctors who are finally speaking up against vaccinations that are mandatory in spite of huge reputational and professional consequences will become a formidable advocate for the elimination.

If a mother-to-be was to ask me if she should follow her doctor's advice to have the flu shot or DaPT, I would advise that if you wish put your baby in an uncontrolled, vast experiment with no informed consent, because tests for safety of the fetus have not been conducted, and cannot legally be done, then definitely. If a parent of a child who is crawling along the street comments that dirt can boost the immune system of their child, I think that this whole meme was based on research that compared the prevalence of autoimmune illnesses for those who are not vaccinated Waldorf students who visited farms during the weekends, non-vaccinated Amish farm kids, "traditional" Swiss farm children, likely more unvaccinated and less vaccinated Brazilian children living in slums against urban kids who are vaccinated. When I witness children being fed harmful waste, or texting on their smartphones sat on top of their children's skulls, I'm shocked, yet I'm not likely to inform them about the lasting harm they're causing to their children, and yet they parents are often the same ones who believe they are entitled to force me to expose my kid to their idea about "health care."

BUILDING AN ALLIANCE FOR REPEAL OF SB277

Parents who exclude their children from vaccinations or defer them through conditions for school entry, are likely to be educated and have higher earnings than those who do not exercise. The best way to combat this is to engage in debate with the herd to defeat the powerful organizations that advocate for mandatory vaccination and form coalitions with unlikely partners to repeal the SB277. We can ultimately demolish the wall of vaccines with precise objectives, skillful tactics and battles that are symmetrical using various strategies.

California citizen petitions to repeal SB277 through a referendum was a challenge to overcome, yet it offered chances to educate those who aren't sure and create a community of support for Freedom of Choice in Health Care. It is a continuous process, however it could be as simple as a message inside the form of a bottle that is floating into a sea of pro-vaxx propagandism.

The lawsuits against Head On struggled to enter the arena and even less achieve the top spot, and were all dismissed by judges who ruled against the state in the year 2017. Fourth lawsuit filed against the California's SB277 was rejected by a federal court this January, despite the fact the law does not violate the federal Constitutional rights of the right of bodily autonomy. This also includes the right to decline unnecessary medical treatment as well as the fundamental right of parents to determine the educational path of their children as well as California the state's constitutional rights to public education.

The judge in the federal court resisted state courts when it came to applying this right. It's a bit like early voter right decisions made in the deep south.Court cases may sometimes break through the veil of media invisibility However, the legal process can be a difficult task and costly.

The Supreme Court granted vaccine manufacturers almost complete immunity from liability back in 2011 and declared that they were "unavoidably unsafe." Based upon their interpretation of 1986 law, they were not liable even if they'd produced a safer vaccination. The gun industry is the only one with immunity similar to the one they enjoy.

The organizations "regulating" them have repeatedly "warned" companies violating manufacturing regulations on contamination without imposing fines or recalling their products, not even ones with glass fragments inside the product. Others contaminants aren't even being checked for. These kinds of friends pharmaceutical corporations that manufacture vaccines aren't in a position to offer safe vaccines, except if they're designed for livestock, and not for the human "herd".

Producers will only be accountable in the case of vaccines for humans if they are aware of injuries that have occurred repeatedly caused by their product and do not make a report to the FDA. If they aren't aware because they haven't asked the FDA, then they're good. As pre-licensing studies only take a couple of days to complete and aren't able to compare placebo-based injections against each other, only post-license research into safety monitoring can reveal what the actual numbers are.

They are not often done due to the fact that they can lead to withdrawals of vaccines. This includes the DPT that caused "high levels of swelling in the arms as well as febrile convulsions, and prolonged times of numbness or limbs that are not responsive. If we do not conduct this research, there'll become more individuals who do not trust in vaccinations. The lack of action results in the credibility of vaccines to decline. It is a loss of credibility" Neal Halsey, a pediatric physician at the Johns Hopkins Bloomberg School of Public Health stated. (The Real Issues in Vaccine Safety,Nature, May 26, 2011)

The most vulnerable chink on the back of totalitarian vaccination is the safety of vaccines. The actual monitoring of injuries can be faulty due to a variety of diagnostics, misreporting and manipulation of the data. Safety of vaccinations suffers due to similar biases in the publication of positive studies on vaccines in general. Insufficient evidence, or a lack of knowledge about the evidence available permits pediatricians to administer toxic shots at night.

Robert Kennedy, Jr. claims he's pro-vaxx however, he is in favor of "safer vaccinations." This is an acceptable middle ground that everyone can agree. After 10 years of pushing for the Food and Drug Administration (FDA) and the Center for Disease Control (CDC) to get rid of the mercury-based preservative Thimerosal used in vaccines, his advocacy led these health departments to request the voluntary elimination of Thimerosal from childhood vaccines back in 2001. (Except for flu vaccines as well as grandfathering in the existing supply of vaccines for children.) The FDA has never acknowledged that mercury is an issue, however they gave Thimerosal's maker all-encompassing immunity via an overnight rider.

It's odd that the National Center for Disease Control's National Immunization Program (NIP) is the one responsible for assessing the safety of the vaccines they've licensed. This is a decision that they have influence over by way of the Advisory Committee on Immunization Practices (ACIP). In order to fulfill their legal obligation in controlling diseases via vaccination, they spend about half of their $11 billion budget for purchasing vaccines, as a part of their mission to boost "uptake.".

The FDA is a statutory authority for vaccination safety, which includes supervision of manufacturing and licensing however, they are not in a position to ensure that the public is confident regarding vaccinations. It's a fact, since they aren't equipped with the resources and autonomy to monitor the safety of vaccines. There are several organizations, including the National Institute of Health, Health Services Resource Administration, Department of Veterans

Affairs and Department of Defense, along with pharmaceutical firms (the producers) and advocacy groups for diseases (their puppets) may play a part in ensuring the safety of vaccines but their main goals are not compatible with the pursuit of the other.

In their responsibilities to supervise the safety of vaccines The Department of Health and Human Services (DHHS) is more involved. The National Vaccine Program Office (NVPO) was initially charged to achieve the highest degree of protection against disease via vaccination and also the least number of vaccine-related adverse reactions. Congress eliminated the entire NVPO funds in 1995 and eliminated their power over CDC as well as the FDA. DHHS is also responsible of advertising vaccines to the general public, and also defending against injuries from vaccines by establishing the Vaccine Injury Compensation Program. (VICP). The VICP is a court that hears instances behind closed doors, supervised with administrative judges from the DHHS. Parents of a affected child will need to engage lawyers and expert witnesses to get past the maze of U.S. Department of Justice barristers who are able to prove the causality.

They are not a good thing at best. Thus, any efforts we make to move the bureaucracies that are adamant about imposing these burdens must focus on exposing their shaky foundations they rely on. In fact, the CDC acknowledges that "public confidence in immunization is critical to sustaining and increasing vaccination coverage rates." The National Research Council of the National Academy of Sciences recommended that the responsibilities of risk assessment and risk management should be divided to increase the confidence of their autonomy. (Much less advertising and purchase). It's not very scientific, but it's still logical.

"It's unlikely that those who recommend a drug for approval could later conduct a dispassionate evaluation of possible harm due to the drug" Public health researchers cited as an FDA critique. They suggested that an Independent National Vaccine Safety Board have the authority to oversee the safety of vaccines and investigate them, as well as the power to recall particular vaccine lines or batches. They were worried about that the reintroduction of smallpox vaccination "because this vaccine causes more serious adverse events than other routinely administered vaccines."

They also offered their services to the National Transportation Safety Board (established in the year 1976 by the Department of Transportation, then declared independent in the year 1975. It was created primarily for the purpose of improving safety in air travel and has. However, it hasn't been as effective in reducing highway crashes up to European standards.) It's "a useful model to ensure optimal vaccine safety and enhance pubic confidence in vaccines."

They called for the adoption "before some real or perceived crisis results in loss of credibility." Their study was disregarded. (Enhancing Public Confidence in Vaccines Through Independent Oversight of Postlicensure Vaccine Safety, American Journal of Public Health, Jan. 2004)

It's a reasonable idea After all, who would have a reason to be against vaccines that are safer or more secure traveling?

"It's very unlikely that vaccine makers are going to remake routine children's vaccines at great cost for no financial benefit", Dr. Paul Offit admitted in his book Vaccinated."Regulatory burdens would be immense," (costing $800 million or more for new vaccines), and they "wouldn't increase sales, only costs. Given that these diseases are rare, it will be hard to run large-scale trials enough to demonstrate that they work."

"Vaccines are natural products. It is impossible to make them completely secure" Juhani Eskola of Finland's National Institute for Healthand Welfare stated. (Nature 5/26/2011) This is, therefore, an attempt to checkmate, not an "flying king" checkers gambit.

In cases where vaccines kill or incapacitate in a way "unfortunate" patients can't sue. They can only request funds via the VICP Private system established in 1986 following expensive civil court rulings were ruled against vaccine makers. Court trials that were open to the public have been damaging profits of vaccines as well as reducing public trust regarding the safety of vaccines. The quantity of "recommended" childhood doses have increased by a third since the introduction of this protection. The funds awarded are not a comfort to the thousands of parents whose kids were hurt or killed due to vaccines. But the compensation for injuries is rarely given.

"Parents who have experienced the grueling, bureaucratic process to prove their cases say the program needs more scrutiny as California and other states tighten their vaccine laws." The Bay Area News Group reported on August 15, 2015 following California Senate Bill 277, which bans medical exemptions from schoolchildren was approved. The law only has the limit of a quarter million dollars in the event of death, the suffering of a patient, however many settlements are lower. Most people don't meet the three-year date to claim due to the fact that their doctor didn't tell the parents about the issue when they asked for medical treatment for the quick reactions.

Brain damage and developmental delay for babies might not be recognized until the deadlines for parents and the victims. However, despite these barriers to compensation more than 16,000 lawsuits have been made since 1987. 10,000 of them were dismissed without any appeal. Since 2005, the bulk of the claimants are adults that were harmed by the influenza vaccines.

The Institute of Medicine (IoM) Immunization Safety Review Committee analyzed the "scientific" literature in 2012 but couldn't come up with sufficient studies that were credible enough to disqualify vaccines that cause 134 of 155 brain, and immune system, or nerve injuries as well as other ailments that were reported by the Vaccine Adverse Event Reporting System (VAERS).

The safety of vaccines is based on untrue information from the VAERS system. The CDC estimates that just 10% of vaccine-related injuries had been reported by medical professionals during 1993, to the VAERS which is administered by the FDA. The FDA has not taken any effective steps to improve mandatory reporting for doctors were enacted over the 25 years to guarantee the safety of vaccines. There isn't any penalty for not reporting. to submit.

The Harvard Pilgrim HMO's internal disclosed vaccine-related reactions were uploaded to VAERS in the year 2010, their rates were 1 out of 10. Add that to the 60,000 that were reported in 2016 with the death of 450, 1,000 permanent impairments as well as 10,000 ER visits, and another half million entries in the base of data since when it was first created.

Neil Miller analyzed the reports of serious injuries to 40,000 and infant deaths in VAERS. He found that they had a higher chance of being injured by more injections (as numerous as eight in a row) and a younger age. Common reactions like asthma, allergy, fevers joint pains and ear infections have not been mentioned. It doesn't even take into account chronic illnesses that develop after many years of numerous vaccinations. This is a huge number of people that do not know why they are in the first place.

The parents of children who are ill with vaccines are among the strongest and hard-working population that is pushed for its removal. They aren't able bear the responsibility, not to mention of their lives already scattered taking care of their children. A lot of parents don't even realize the dangers of vaccines and how they kill due to corporate media control. Parents are looking for answers. That's the reason Senator. Dick Pan, the SB277 patron, is seeking to stop the independent media outlets that sell "fake news", read vaxx-truther sites.

Vaccine Security is the criterion that will be pushed further with each physician's appointment. If they mention vaccines be sure to ask regarding VAERS, and how they are familiar in reporting. Any possible future payment either for yourself or your child is contingent on the prompt reporting of any injuries.

Another force that could be a formidable one could be the wounded veterans of the military who were harmed due to mandatory vaccinations received without consent or informed consent or even a consent form once they joined the military. The source of this isn't either the Veterans Administration or the Defense Department due to their ties with the CDC, DHHS, IoM and FDA. Our comrades can be seen at Veterans of Foreign Wars and American Legion halls and they will be angry, but without being able to decide who they should be mad with.

When Bart Classen, M.D. presented evidence in Congress U.S. Congress that mandatory vaccination for soldiers increase the incidence of insulin-dependent diabetes by about 25 percent, he also criticized the anthrax vaccine specifically that is "not properly tested and likely to cause problems", that was compounded when it was combined with DPT vaccine. He predicted it will increase immune-mediated diseases when administered to people who are adults. Gulf War Syndrome is still not considered a vaccine-related injury yet it does have many hallmarks.His findings were criticized from The Department of Defense. He accuses U.S. Public Health Service of "acting like propaganda officers to support political agendas" in providing false information. Invite the vets to join the fold and let them make their point.

Certain allies do not doubt the efficacy of vaccinations and are in opposition to different aspects of mandatory vaccination. The Catholic Church as well as pro-life Christians will be shocked and at first, when confronted with abortion-related embryonic cells as part of some compulsory vaccines. The spontaneous abortions that vaccines cause pregnant women, as well as an increase in mortality of babies.

Certain religious organizations are unhappy with their presence with philosophical exceptions However, this is an issue that's bipartisan that should be limited to edges. Freedom of Choice isn't a either a conservative or liberal issue. All legislators who supported prohibiting parental choices on the state of California were Democrat however, they were Republican or moderate Democrat within Mississippi.

Do not insult or provoke during your discussions However, be sure to take part in a civilized debate. Make sure you are the logical one present since we have already earned been branded as batshit insane. Being respectful of our adversaries as well as allies beliefs or systems of non-belief will help to form those unbreakable connections that are required to stop this monster from escaping. The ones who are most opposed could end up being the fiercest advocates once they realise how liars they had been.

A few allies could be people who are libertarian-leaning and have no children, who think they are not interested playing the game. They're utterly wrong and must be reminded of the laws being developed to require people working in the fields of health care, senior services, and child care facilities to get vaccinated. These categories could be extended until there's none that isn't. There are more than 200 vaccines that are in the pipeline, all waiting to be included in the list.

School officials may be convinced by financial reasons if sufficient parents are against totalitarian rules which cost them money as well as time with the strategies described in the previous chapter. It's more expensive and time consuming for school districts to provideIndividualized Education Plansdue to diagnoseddisabilities. The children may be exempt by federal laws that guarantee their rights for equal education access.

Chapter 5: What Is Polio?

Following the World Health Assembly passed a resolution calling for the elimination of polio across the world and the Global Polio Eradication Initiative (GPEI) was established, which was led by the government officials from each country, WHO, Rotary International and The US Centers for Disease Control and Prevention (CDC), as well as UNICEF it was established in the year 1988. Then, in the following years in the year, the GPEI was added to by Bill & Melinda Gates Foundation as well as Gavi as which is the Vaccine Alliance. After the demise of smallpox around 1980 the incidence of polio is down 99percent globally over the time of its elimination, and the condition that can affect the majority of people has been eliminated.

An estimated 350 000 cases spread across over the 125 countries that were endemic from 1988, to just 6 cases by 2021, there's been fewer than one percent instances of wild poliovirus reported in the years since the year 1988.

The year 1952 saw the total number of polio-related cases within the United States reached a peak of 57,000 instances. There has been no cases of polio anywhere in any of the United States since the Polio Vaccination Assistance Act was introduced in the year 1982.

While many countries have earned the same certificate however, polio is evident in some countries that haven't launched vaccination programs. WHO Trusted Source states that since there's been an unconfirmed incident of polio, kids all over the world are at risk.

The immunization campaign in Afghanistan is scheduled to commence in October or even early November of this year. There are current and coming national and subnational immunization Day across the continent in West Africa.

Because of the fear and widespread response to diseases There was an incredible mass mobilization, which led to developing cutting-edge techniques to prevent and treat illness in addition to making medical aid revolutionary. Poliomyelitis's impact is present in the design of new rehabilitation therapies as well as the global expansion of disability rights organisations, in spite of the elimination of wild poliomyelitis across only two countries (Afghanistan and Pakistan)[3][44.

The virus that triggers the highly infectious illness polio (also called poliomyelitis) can affect your nervous system. The children who are younger than five are more susceptible to contracting the disease more than other.

But, due to the worldwide eradication campaign that began in 1988, these regions were declared as polio-free

Americas, Southeast Asia, and the Western Pacific

The polio vaccine was first developed in the year 1953, and made accessible in the year 1957. Since then, there's seen fewer cases of polio the US.

Yet, polio remains within Afghanistan, Pakistan, and Nigeria. Medically and economically, the elimination of polio is beneficial to everyone around the globe. The elimination of polio could result in savings of between $40 and $50 billion in the coming 20 years.

Information that is important

Most cases of polio (poliomyelitis) cases are involving young children who are less than five.

The condition of paralysis is not repaired after 200 infections. In the event that their respiratory muscles are inactive, 5 to 10 percentage of people that are disabled die.

There were only six cases of poliovirus wild reported in the years since 1988. This is compared with the estimated 350 000 cases reported at the time.

If there's a single sick child, polio is an issue for children across the world. If polio can't be eliminated from the last major strongholds it could be the case that there is a global spread of the illness.

The efforts of the world have helped countries improve their ability to tackle other infectious diseases through the establishment of efficient surveillance and vaccination systems.

What are the Signs of polio

There is a good chance that 95-99 percent of the people suffering from poliovirus do not show any symptoms. It is a condition known as subclinical or undetected polio. Although they may not show any symptoms, individuals with poliovirus could be infected and transmit it to people around them.

Non-paralytic Polio

From one to ten days, polio-like symptoms that are not paralytic and symptoms may continue. Meningitis, fevers, a headache, sore throat fatigue, nausea and fatigue are only a few of the flu-like symptoms and symptoms that could manifest.

Polio that is not paralytically caused is commonly called abortion or polio.

The paralysis caused by polio

About 1% of the polio-related infections can cause paralysis. The brainstem is paralyzed as well as the spinal cord both are caused through paralytic Polio (spinal paralytic polio) (bulb spine polio).

The first signs of non-paralytic the disease are identical in a variety of instances. But, symptoms will get worse over the course of one period of one week. Temporary or even permanent weakness; loss of reflexes painful muscle spasms; drooping or slack legs, usually on one side and limbs with deformities including the hips feet and ankles are just a few signs.

Paralysis in complete form is very common. It is estimated that only 1% of cases of polio can be able to cause permanent impairment in accordance with an independent source. Within 5-10% of instances that suffer from polio paralysis virus can attack muscles responsible for breathing. It can end in the death of.

Poliomyelitis-related syndrome

The disease can recur after recovery. It can happen within 15 to 40 years after. PPS (post-polio syndrome) (PPS) symptoms are chronic joint and muscular weakening, a rise in muscle pain and fatigue, restlessness or easy and muscle atrophy. It can also cause difficulty breathing and swallowing difficulties, sleep apnea or breathing problems related to sleep as well as a decrease in tolerance to cold temperatures, as well as depression.

Troubles with concentration and memory

See your physician if you were a victim of polio but are experiencing these signs. PPS is a common occurrence in 25 to 50 percent of those who have survived polio, according to research. It is not transmitted to those suffering from the disease. The treatment involves a variety of measures that increase your overall quality of life and reduce fatigue or discomfort.

A doctor will be able to determine the presence of polio through studying your symptoms. The doctor will conduct an examination of your body, searching for issues such as weak reflexes, stiffness of the back and neck or difficulty in raising your head while lying on the floor.

Furthermore, laboratories will analyze the cerebrospinal fluid, feces or the throat for evidence of Poliovirus.

Eradication

Once they are properly implemented, strategies for eradicating polio are successful. The fact that the disease is now eradicated successfully across the vast majority of countries around the world proves the fact.

The Polio Eradication Strategy 2022-2026 outlines the steps to ensure the world from viruses that cause polio for the rest of time in the meantime, as well as continuous shift and post-certification initiatives are underway to ensure that the framework established to eliminate the disease will be able to support other initiatives in public health long after the disease is eliminated.

ensuring that the Strategy is well-funded and carried out across the entire spectrum is vital to achieve the success. Failure to implement strategies can lead to continued spread of the virus. The wild poliovirus virus continues to be throughout Afghanistan as well as Pakistan. Failure to end polio these areas could result in a global recurrence of the disease. In this regard, it is essential to ensure that polio is always eradicated.

Once polio has been removed, everyone can celebrate the accomplishment of a major world-wide public good that can all people equally, regardless of the place they live. Based on economic models that polio elimination will yield savings of around USaround $40 to $50 billion mostly in the developing countries. The most important thing is that it will ensure that future generations of children are not from the dreadful effects of permanent paralysis caused by polio.

In accordance with the International Health Regulations, the international campaign for the elimination of the polio virus has been classified as an Public Health Initiative of International Concern as well as interim recommendations are being offered to nations who suffer from poliovirus or have a high likelihood of the disease returning.

The polio campaign continues in support of more extensive public health initiatives by providing monitoring of disease to support larger public health initiatives and responding to natural catastrophes such as humanitarian disasters and earthquakes. and other outbreaks of infections. The GPEI continues to provide assistance to the COVID-19 response, including support for monitoring disease levels lab capacity and the development of vaccines and distribution.

Chapter 6: What Is The Transmission Route For Polio

In the wake of the finding of probable communicable poliovirus transmission in the course of regular surveillance at London, British health authorities have declared a national emergency. Stephen Sosler, Head of Vaccine Programs at Gavi, talks to Linda Geddes how this might be the case.

The oral-oral (or the source of pharyngeal infection) as well as the fecal-oral (intestinal source) methods of transmission the poliomyelitis virus are extremely infectious.

Polioviruses that are wild can infect nearly all human beings in areas where they're prevalent. In climates with temperate temperatures where transmission is highest, it occurs during the autumn and summer. In tropical areas, there are more subtle seasonal changes. Incubation time, referred to as the period between the initial exposure and beginning of symptoms, usually runs between 6 to 20 days. It can be extended to a time of 3 to 35 days. After a few weeks of initial infection, viruses are eliminated through excreted feces. Drinking or eating food that is contaminated is the primary way this illness spreads through the fecal-oral route. The virus can also be transmitted orally to a person else, which is prevalent in environments where hygiene and sanitation are in good condition. While transmission is possible when the virus is in saliva or feces and feces, the virus is more likely to spread within 7-10 days of and following the appearance of symptoms. Insufficiency in immunity, malnutrition or physical activity immediately following the onset of weakness, damage to skeletal muscles caused by the injection of vaccinations or therapeutic agents, as well as the pregnancy of a child are all factors that increase the risk of contracting polio, or affect on the extent of illness. The fetus is not believed to be affected by mother's illness or the polio vaccine however it is possible that the virus will pass through over the barrier between mother and child in the course of the course of pregnancy. In the initial few days of the baby's life the passive immunity given by antibodies from the mother and cross-resistance to the placenta, shields the baby from getting the polio virus.

If a person suffering from polio is coughing or sneezing or gets in contact with excrement, the illness is spread (fecal-oral method).

Do not wash your hands following use of the bathroom or dealing with feces in two methods of spreading (like change of diapers).

• Injecting water that is contaminated into your mouth, or drinking it.

Food that has been exposed to contaminated water.

Swimming in polluted water. If someone suffering from diarrhea bathes in the waters, it is possible that the water will become polluted.

coughing up or sniffing.

Living in close proximity to someone suffering from polio.

Avoiding the polluted surface.

The polio virus is usually spread through hands that been in contact with an infected person's urine to the mouth, from where it is absorbed into the body. Also, there could be oral-tooral and respiratory transmission via saliva. It could take as long as 30 days for the flu like mild symptoms to appear (fatigue or fever, headache muscle pain, stiffness nausea) in which period the patient may spread the virus to people around them.

Polio can spread more easily in areas that have lower vaccination rates. Every New Yorker aged 2 months and over must receive the vaccine against polio as fast as is possible due to this.

PREGNANCY, FETUS, AND NEWBORN POLIOMYELITIS

A 20-year-old woman discovered she had acute anterior poliomyelitis during the autumn of 1954. She was pregnant, and the question was whether the fetus was affected prior to or following the birth. The question of whether she was allowed to utilize the maternity services and also the infant nursery at the hospital nearby was also raised nine days following the diagnosis when labor began. As the mother had finished the California state's seven-day isolation requirements, her access was judged as relatively secure.

A baby boy was not injured. Poliomyelitis afflicted this baby the second day of his the baby's life. Gammaglobulin was given to 11 more babies in the nursery in the same day.

The study did not reveal any other cases that could be observed.

POLIOMYELITIS in the course of GRANDMOTHER Pregnancy is believed to increase the likelihood of developing and the occurrence of paralytic. Fox, Sennett, and Waaler collected 95 cases where it was feasible to make a precise comparison against the females with no gravid populace.

Polio vaccines

What are the functions of vaccinations?

As we walk around and in our bodies bacteria are everywhere. An infectious organism can cause the death of a person if it gets into contact with an insecure person.

The body's system has a myriad of defense mechanisms to guard its body from infection (disease-causing bacteria). Physical barriers like mucus, skin and the cilia (tiny hairs which carry substances away from the lung) are all designed to prevent infections from ever reaching the body.

In the event that a virus invades the body The immune system of the body gets activated and the infection is attacked by the body, and is either eliminated or defeated.

The normal reaction of the body

A virus, bacterium parasite, fungus, or other that can cause body and cause illness is known as an agent of pathogen. Every pathogen is comprised of many smaller elements which are usually exclusive to the specific pathogen and the disease it can cause. The antigen is the part of a pathogen, which triggers the creation of antibodies. The most important element of the immune system are the antigens produced in response to the antigen that causes the disease. The concept of antibodies can be described as soldiers in the body's defense mechanism. Each and every antibody that we produce is a soldier who is trained to recognize specific antigens. Our bodies are stocked with a variety of antibodies. It takes an amount of time for your immune system create antibodies that target an antigen when your body first comes in contact to it.

A person is also susceptible to getting sick during the time.

When they're created, antigen specific antibodies are able to interact with other components part of our immune system in order to remove the pathogen, and stop the disease. In rare cases, if two viruses have a lot of similarities in their respective ways like family members, antibodies against the same pathogen are usually not able to defend against the other. Alongside the production of antibodies in the course of an initial response towards an antigen, the body also creates memories cells that produce antibodies even after the pathogen is removed by the antibodies. Since the memory cells are able to make antibodies against the specific antigen, in the event that your body has to be confronted with the same illness multiple times it will produce antibodies stronger and faster than the initial time around.

Then, in the event that someone is infected with the infection that is harmful the body's immune system is able to respond quickly, thus avoiding disease.

Antigens are the components of an organism (antigen) that trigger an immune-related reaction in the body. They are present in vaccinations. As opposed to the actual antigen the most recent vaccines contain their recipe to make the antigen. No matter if the vaccine comprises an antigen in itself or instructions that the body must follow to produce the antigen this less potent form will not make the person sick. Instead it can trigger the body's immune system to act in the same way it did as a response to the pathogen.

Certain vaccinations require multiple doses that are spaced out several weeks or months. Sometimes, it is essential for the development of memory cells as well as the creation of long-lasting antibodies. When you develop memory of the pathogen, your body is able to fight the specific disease-causing organism which allows it to rapidly respond to any subsequent encounters.

Group immunity

One who is given the vaccination is probably being protected from the disease being at risk. However, not all people are eligible to receive a vaccination. Certain vaccines might not be appropriate for individuals to take when they are sensitive to one or more vaccine elements or have medical conditions that affect their immune system (such for example, cancer and HIV). If those individuals are living with or are among those who've had vaccinations, they might have been safe. If a significant part of the population has been vaccination-free, the virus will have an extremely difficult time spreading because many of the people they come in contact with are protected. Thus, the greater number of people that are protected from the virus more likely the people that aren't of being ever exposed to the harmful diseases. The term is called herd immunity.

It is essential for those who are not able to receive vaccinations but are also susceptible to illnesses that which we are immunized against. Herd immunity doesn't completely safeguard those who aren't adequately immunized. In fact, there is no vaccine that can provide the complete security. With herd immunity, people who have herd immunity will be protected in a significant way. security since other people around them have had vaccinations.

The benefits of getting vaccinated go beyond protecting the individual, but it also assists those living in communities who are unable to receive vaccinations. You should consider getting your vaccine if have the chance.

Humans have developed vaccines all over the world for a wide range of dangerous diseases, such as measles, tetanus and meningitis and wild Poliovirus.

In the entire world at the first decade of the 20th century, polio crippled millions of people every year. Two effective vaccines to combat the disease had been developed in the year 1950. But, the vaccinations were not widespread enough in some regions of the world, including Africa in order to prevent the spread of the polio virus. A global effort to remove polio from globe began in the late 1980s. The vaccination of polio has been carried out on every continent over several years, and decades of frequent vaccinations and massive vaccination programmes. The African continent has been declared free of wild poliovirus in the month of August, 2020. It has joined every other region of the globe, with the notable one exception: Pakistan and Afghanistan in which polio has not yet been completely eradicated due to vaccination of thousands of people, primarily youngsters.

Although the disease is mostly present only in Afghanistan and Pakistan today however, it was a severe child illness that afflicted people around the globe throughout the latter half of 19th and 20th century. Even though it was commonplace to receive polio vaccines by the 1970s that significantly reduced the incidence of the disease but by the mid-80s it was still crippling over 1,000 kids per daily.

The Global Polio Eradication Initiative (GPEI) that in that Gavi is a part founded in 1988. The initiative was a major influence in the fight against this disease. It brought together the governments and local communities, donors as well as health professionals, working together to educate the public about the illness and to increase accessibility to vaccines against polio.

Many countries now have zero cases following a dramatic reduction in cases which was observed over the past 100 percent. Since the beginning of GPEI, around 20 million kids are protected from getting the disease. This was an important achievement in the year Nigeria was declared to be free of wild poliovirus, in the year 2020 because it was among the countries that had been spared of the disease had remained.

The vaccine can aid people in developing poliovirus resistance. There are two varieties of poliovirus vaccinations that are available for oral administration: attenuated orally administered poliovirus and inactivated poliovirus administered by injectable (IPV) (OPV). IgG as well as IgM antibodies, created after receiving the polio vaccine, could prevent the spread of the virus to motor neuron cells in the nervous system's central part. Antibodies also are present in the tonsils as well as the gastrointestinal tract following vaccination.

Polio vaccines are vaccinations that serve to protect against from poliomyelitis (polio).

Inactivated poliovirus (IPV) is given intravenously. Meanwhile, the less weakened poliovirus is administered by mouth (OPV).

The World Health Organization (WHO) suggests that children receive all polio vaccines.

The vast majority of the world is free of the disease thanks to the two vaccines. It has also decreased the number of reported cases by 350,000 from 1988 to only 33 cases in the year 2018.

The polio vaccines are completely inactivated and highly secured.

The site of injection may show small amounts of redness, or even soreness.

For every million doses of vaccine administered the oral polio vaccination results in three cases of vaccine-associated paralytic poliomyelitis.

The figure is in contrast to 5,000 cases per million people becoming disabled after contracting polio.

The two forms of vaccine are generally appropriate for use by expectant mothers, as well as HIV/AIDS patients who are otherwise in good health.

New oral polio vaccine types 2 (nOPV2) is a plan to improve the safety of the vaccine and thus prevent the recurrence of the circulating vaccine-derived poliovirus (cVDPV), which is a variant in the vaccine virus which has recurred to cause poliomyelitis is triggered due to the outbreak of cVDPV.

Hilary Koprowski made the first successful demonstration of polio vaccination in 1950 with a drinkable attenuated virus.

While the vaccine was utilized efficiently in Europe however, it was not approved to be used for use in the United States. In 1955, Jonas ' activated (killed) the polio vaccine classified as successful. Albert Sabin created a second live oral polio vaccine with a lower toxicity and it was made available for use in clinical trials in the year 1961.

Despite the extraordinary magnitude of these successes experts from polio warn that further progress needs to be made prior to the time when the disease has been completely eliminated. If the global climate changes and infectious diseases that have been virtually eliminated could recur with surprising ease. Measles, for instance, are beginning to increase because of the decline in vaccination rates across Europe as well as the US. COVID-19's effect on the regular vaccination schedule worldwide and the uneven global coverage of polio vaccines which has resulted in measles outbreaks in previously undiscovered regions. A rash of cases was reported in Ukraine during the month of October in 2021 followed by Malawi discovered a case wild the poliovirus virus in February 2022. In Pakistan which is where the disease remains prevalent there were more cases of polio discovered in the early 30 days of 2022 than the entire 2021 period. In March, polio caused by vaccines was detected in Israel.

Although polio is only affecting the countries of a tiny percentage currently and is not a major threat to the world at present, there is a reason why the World Health Organization still considers the disease to be considered a Public Health Emergency of International Concern (PHEIC) regardless the fact that this declaration was issued earlier in the year 2014.

An ancient illness

One of the oldest diseases that exists in the world is polio. Illustrations dating back to 14th century Egypt depict a priest who had legs that are swollen, which is one of the most distinctive features of the condition. It can cripple the limb, causing the muscles to weaken and shrink. The first clinical explanation of the disease was published in 1789 by British physician Michael Underwood. Doctor. Jacob Von Heine, an expert German orthopedist, understood the fact that poliomyelitis is a disease that was distinct from other forms of paralysis. He believed that it was caused by an infectious cause in 1840. Austrian physician Karl Landsteiner first isolated the virus that causes poliomyelitis in 1909.

Highly contagious disease that can be spread through unhygienic practices or through drinking contaminated food or drinks. It is most often found in areas that are not able to access sanitary sanitation facilities as well as clean water.

Vaccine creation

There are two varieties of polio vaccines. One is the live attenuated oral polio vaccination (OPV) which was developed by Dr. Albert Sabin in 1961 and inactivated (killed) vaccination against polio (IPV) developed by Dr. Jonas Salk in 1955.

IPV can be injected as a vaccination that is made of inactivated wild-type Poliovirus strains of all kinds. In a number of countries, it's given along with other routine immunizations for children like diphtheria pertussis, and tetanus.

The live poliovirus strains attenuated which comprise OPV consist from each of the three serotypes. Though it's reliable and safe, application of OPV in regions with inadequate sanitation and water can result in an unwanted side effect. There are rare occasions where the virus that is shed live by people who have been vaccinated can change and then spread to populations where polio has not completely eradicated.

In the longer that the virus resulting by a vaccine can spread and spread, the lower the level of immune system. The strain is known as the circulating vaccine-derived poliovirus can sometimes regain its ability to cause damage to the nervous system, causing involuntary paralysis (cVDPV).

While IPV is an excellent vaccine, and is useful for countries that do not have a polio epidemic but it's best used to prevent the spread of polio as it is not able to create the same immune response like OPV and therefore is less effective in stopping the propagation of poliovirus live. The primary place that virus replicates, which is the stomach, is in the gut, where OPV boosts mucosal immunity. In turn, the vaccine prevents the spread of poliovirus in the surrounding environment. It can limit or stop transmission. This is essential in areas that are more prone to come in contact with infections caused by water, for instance areas that have inadequate water or sanitation.

So, OPV continues to be mandatory in those areas that require transmission to be stopped, even though IPV was added into routine immunization programmes within Gavi-supported nations.

The oral vaccination against polio (nOPV2) is a vaccine that is developed to be genetically more stable than the Sabin variant and less likely to trigger instances due to vaccine-derived virus. It is a new weapon to the arsenal.

In order to facilitate a rapid launch, nOPV2 was granted the approval of the World Health Organization's Emergency Use Listing (EUL) protocol in November. There are 20 countries included in the list, which includes Benin, Cameroon, Congo, Djibouti, Egypt, Ethiopia, The Gambia, Guinea-Bissau Liberia, Mauritania, Mozambique, Niger, Nigeria, Senegal, Sierra Leone, Tajikistan and Uganda and has administered nearly 350 million doses of NOPV2 by June 2022.

But, the GPEI seeks to reduce an issue of supply that is caused from the intense need for this vaccination. A trivalent oral vaccine against polio (tOPV) could be the most effective method of immunization when there is co-circulation between the poliovirus strains according to the GPEI.

Two of the endemic countries confront significant challenges in the fight to eliminate the disease of polio. In Pakistan it is still difficulties in reaching the high-risk mobile populations, caused due to the fact that some areas of the country have low coverage of routine vaccinations as well as parents who are hesitant to vaccine their children because of inexperience or simply because of community fatigue.

A lot of the issues mentioned such as vaccine hesitancy are present within Afghanistan and elsewhere, where years of instability and violence have damaged the health care system and stopped the government from promoting regular vaccinations. The children are at risk to contract polio as a consequence of under- or insufficient vaccinations of many populations.

To combat false information and to increase awareness of how important it is to get vaccination, efforts to eradicate have been intensified as polio vaccination programs returned. This could mean enlisting the assistance of local and religious leaders, as well as expanding the supply of vaccines to improve vaccination coverage.

Chapter 7: Vaccines

It is biochemical formulation that increases the immunity of an illness. It typically has something that is similar to an organism that is responsible for causing disease. It's typically made of weak or dead varieties of the microbe, the toxins it produces or its proteins on the surface. The substance stimulates your body's immune system to identify it as foreign, remove it and create an account of the event, to ensure that your immune system is able to be more readily recognize and eradicate the microorganisms they later come across.

Developing Immunity

The immune system recognizes agents as a foreign invader, kills the virus, then "remembers" them. If the virus version of an agent comes into contact and the body detects the protein coat that covers the virus. It will be prepared to fight it through (1) neutralizing targeted agent prior to it entering cells as well as (2) the body recognizes and destroys the infected cells prior to when that virus is able to multiply into huge quantities.

Vaccines have helped in the elimination of smallpox among the more infectious and deadly illnesses known to mankind. Other infections like measles, rubella and polio Mumps, chickenpox and typhoid are not the same as they were years before. In the event that the majority of people are being vaccinated this makes it very difficult for an outbreak to develop, let alone propagate. This is known as herd immunity. Polio, which can be transmitted by humans only, is at the center of an extensive elimination campaign, which has led to the spread of polio to just regions of four nations (Afghanistan, India, Nigeria as well as Pakistan). The difficulties of reaching all children and the cultural differences, however, has caused the expected day of eradication to go by numerous times.

Jonas Salk & the Polio Vaccine

Jonas Edward Salk (October 28 1914 - June 23 1995) was an American doctoral researcher and Virolologist. Salk was the one who discovered and invented the first vaccination against polio that was inactivated. The man was raised in New York City to Jewish parents. Even though they did not have formal training, they wanted to see their children achieve. As a student at New York University School of Medicine, Salk stood out among his classmates, and not only because of his academic achievements however, but also because he opted to go into research in medical science instead of becoming a doctor.

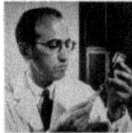

Jonas Salk

Magazine photo, 1956

Born	October 28, 1914 New York, New York
Died	June 23, 1995 (aged 80) La Jolla, California, United States
Residence	New York, New York Pittsburgh, Pennsylvania La Jolla, California
Nationality	American
Fields	Medical research, virology and epidemiology

Up until 1957, when Salk vaccine was introduced in the year 1957, it was thought to be as the most terrifying health threat facing the postwar United States. The annual polio epidemics became increasingly destructive. In 1952, the epidemic was considered to be the most severe outbreak in country's recent past. In the nearly 58,000 cases that were reported during the year, 3,145 passed away and 21,269 suffering from mild to severe paralysis. The majority of the victims were youngsters. People living in urban areas felt frightened each summer as the possibility of recurrence of polio returned.

In an documentary from 2009 PBS document "Apart from the atomic bomb, America's greatest fear was polio." In the aftermath, researchers had to race to discover a method to ward off or eliminate the condition. U.S. president Franklin D. Roosevelt was considered to be the most famous sufferer of the disease. He created the foundation, called the March of Dimes Foundation, to fund research and development of an effective vaccine.

After 1947, Salk took up an offer to join The University of Pittsburgh School of Medicine. He embarked on an initiative that was funded from the National Foundation for Infantile Paralysis to identify the prevalence of polio types. virus. Salk was intrigued by the possibility to further develop this work to develop a vaccine for the polio virus, and along with the highly skilled team of researchers he put together dedicated himself to this research for seven years. The field study established for the purpose of testing Salk's vaccine Salk vaccine was one of the most complex study of its kind ever conducted ever, with more than 20,000 doctors and health professionals, 64,000 teachers and staff, and 220,000 people who participated." More than 1,800,000 pupils participated in the test. The it was announced that the vaccine's effectiveness was announced in April of 1955 Salk was described as an "miracle performer," and the day "almost became a holiday for the entire nation." Salk's sole goal was to create a secure and efficient vaccine as quickly as he could, without desire to make a profit for himself. When asked during a live interview about who held the patent on the vaccine Salk responded: "There is no patent. Could you patent the sun?"

In the year 1960, he established in 1960 the Salk Institute for Biological Studies located in La Jolla, California, it is a place for scientific and medical research. Salk continued conducting studies. Salk's last few days were spent in search of an effective vaccine for HIV. The personal papers of Salk are kept in the University of California, San Diego Library.

Misinformation

False information (from any sources) could create a swarm of distrust and suspicion.

The misinformation process also includes the deliberate diffusion of misleading facts. It is the case that individuals aren't just uncertain about the safety of vaccines, but could be completely opposed to vaccinations.

Untruths about vaccinations are often seen all over the Internet. Certain websites, like do not support the vaccination of children and infants. They make a range of assertions that are generally in contradiction to peer-reviewed science literature.

Misinformation websites tend to rely on emotionally-filled anecdotes about bad things that happened to children or were first recognized--coincidental in time with vaccine administration--while ignoring or distorting scientific studies.

Unfortunately for many communities, anti-vaccine movement have caused harm to the health of people over the years. A study, for instance revealed that anti-vaccine movements the whooping-cough vaccine have caused whooping-cough epidemics across several nations (countries that are just an hour's flight far away).

What can you do to distinguish reliable facts from false information? The most common misinformation is any of the following components:

Invalid Assumptions

Untrue assumptions are those that is treated as if it could be proven to be accurate or untrue, despite the reality, it's not. Some parents, for instance, consider the hepatitis B vaccination as unneeded as if it were a condition in which their children do not stand a danger. It is a false assumption.

Logical Fallacies

Logical fallacies are an inconsistency or flaw that renders an argument incoherent or ineffective. Common logical errors include the ad hominem argument (attacking people who are who are presenting the argument, rather than the argument the argument itself) and appeals to sympathy (trying to convince people to support your arguments through appeals to guilt or sympathy) Arguments based on ignorance (claiming that an assertion is valid only since it hasn't been proved to be false, or the statement is not true because it isn't proved to be valid) and many more.

Ad Hoc Hypotheses

Ad (literally, "for this") (literally, "for this") hypothesis is a modification that is made to a particular theory to keep the theory from being questioned. Ad hoc explanations attempt to clarify observations that are not in line with the theory originally proposed.

False Experts or Experts Who Lack the Needed Expertise

Experts in one particular field could be totally ignorant of an entirely different field. A specialist endocrinologist could be an expert regarding diabetes, however they are not necessarily an authority in the safety of vaccines or about the field of immunology. Unfortunately, those who might have expertise in one area will make bold claims regarding things that are not in their area of competence.

Pseudoscience

The pseudoscientific claims can't be confirmed by any other researcher since they're often unclear and cannot be quantified. The majority of times, the assertions aren't subjected under peer scrutiny (that is, a review conducted by experts) before they are made public and, as such, the procedures are complicated to comprehend, making these observations hard to reproduce. Sometimes, the data could be depicted to indicate one thing but the reality is that it's not. In other instances, the strategies employed are most more likely to result in a predetermined result. Data that supports the claims are presented, whereas other data that contradict the claim are either dismissed or ignored.

Claims	Facts
Natural methods of enhancing immunity are better than vaccinations.	The only "natural way" to be immune is to have the disease. Immunity from a preventive vaccine provides protection against disease when a person is exposed to it in the future. That immunity is usually similar to what is acquired from natural infection, although several doses of a vaccine may have to be given for a child to have a full immune response.
Epidemiology—often used to establish vaccine safety—is not science but number crunching.	Epidemiology is a well-established scientific discipline that, among other things, identifies the cause of diseases and the factors that increase a person's risk for a disease.
Giving multiple vaccines at the same time causes an "overload" of the immune system.	Vaccination does not overburden a child's immune system; the recommended vaccines use only a small portion of the immune system's "memory".
Vaccines are ineffective.	Vaccines have spared millions of people the effects of devastating diseases. (See Vaccine effectiveness).

Common Claims Found on Misinformation Websites

Chapter 8: Childhood Contagious Diseases
Children's immune systems have developed and often live located in close proximity with the other in day care facilities, classrooms, as well as in school busses. This can make the spread of diseases that are contagious particularly simple and helps explain, for a large extent, why illnesses are very common among children. Most contagious illnesses are brought on by the transmission of bacterial (such as those in Scarlet fever) or virus (such as chickenpox, measles, and quite handful of other cases) through droplets of mucus or saliva in particular when one is coughing or sniffing. The majority of contagious diseases can be caused by close contact with an suffering from the disease or exchanging personal belongings of someone who has been infected like in infections caused by parasites (such such as lice and Scabies) or fungal infections (such as tinea infections which is commonly referred to as "ringworm").

The good news is that many childhood diseases when contracted can lead to a life-long immune system in the child who is infected. However, this isn't often the case. The vaccinations also protect against the most contagious illnesses. The chickenpox virus, for instance, is less common as it was just 15 years ago. It usually mild when infected by a child who is vaccinated against chickenpox.

A lot of illnesses are more contagious prior to when the affected child shows any signs or symptoms and, therefore, transmission is higher among kids. The most common changes to the skin occur at a certain stage one of the diseases listed below and can assist in distinguishing among the various contagious childhood conditions and assist you to determine when and whether to contact your child's medical professional.

The list of images below depicting childhood disease transmission is in no way, complete be aware that the majority of these illnesses are avoidable by following the recommended vaccine protocol

Erythema infectiosum, sometimes referred to as Slapped-cheek disease is a prevalent illness that affects youngsters due to the infection of parvovirus B19. The disease can be spread through contacts with other people who are affected.

Roseola Exanthem subitum as well as roseola infantum is a minor illness which mostly affects children and disappears completely on its own. Roseola is due to viruses that are herpes-like.

Measles (Rubeola) is a transmissible infection of the respiratory system that originates from an infection caused by a virus. It isn't a common occurrence within the United States, since immunizations are required since the 1960s.

It is a common occurrence for people to contract chickenpox. (Varicella) is a infection due to the varicella virus, which goes away completely on its own. The virus spreads to humans via respiratory fluids, like coughing, or sneezing.

Scarlet Fever is an infection that is caused by a kind of bacterium known as Streptococcus. This bacteria is not the only cause of an infection of the throat ("strep throat") however, it also creates a poison (toxin) which causes a distinctive itchy rash.

German measles (rubella) originates from the virus rubella. It can be transmitted among people through contact with the fluids of those affected.

Delivery Systems for Vaccinations

There are many innovative delivery methods in the works to make vaccines more effective to distribute.

Recent advances in the field of vaccine delivery has led to oral vaccines. The polio vaccine was created and validated by volunteers without formal education; The results showed that the convenience of vaccines improved. When a vaccine is administered orally the risk is zero from blood contamination. The oral vaccines will be solid and proved to be more durable and less likely to be frozen and this reduces the necessity to have an "cold chain" (the resources necessary to ensure that vaccines are kept within a certain temperature band from the production phase until the time of administration. This, could, in turn, reduce cost of vaccinations).

Microneedles currently in the early stages of development, employs "pointed projections fabricated into arrays that can create vaccine delivery pathways through the skin".

Nanopatch is a injection system without needles which is in the process of being developed. A patch of the size of the adhesive bandage has around 20000 microscopic projections in one square inch. when worn over the skin, it can deliver the vaccine directly onto the skin. It is more populated with immune cells than the muscles in which needles and syringes distribute. This increases the efficacy of vaccination by with a lesser dose of the vaccine that is used in traditional syringe-based delivery systems.

Recommended CDC Vaccinations

In the event that you are behind or begin late in the below schedule for vaccinations the catch-up vaccines must be administered as soon as possible:

Birth to 15 Months

Vaccine	Birth	1 mo	2 mos	4 mos	6 mos	9 mos	12 mos	15 mos
Hepatitis B[1] (HepB)	←1st dose→	←2nd dose→			←3rd dose→			
Rotavirus[2] (RV) RV1 (2-dose series); RV5 (3-dose series)			←1st dose→	←2nd dose→				
Diphtheria, tetanus, & acellular pertussis[3] (DTaP: <7 yrs)			←1st dose→	←2nd dose→	←3rd dose→			←4th dose→
Tetanus, diphtheria, & acellular pertussis[4] (Tdap: ≥7 yrs)								
Type b[5] (Hib) flu vaccine			←1st dose→	←2nd dose→			←3rd or 4th dose	
Pneumococcal conjugate[6] (PCV13)			←1st dose→	←2nd dose→	←3rd dose→		←4th dose→	
Pneumococcal polysaccharide[6] (PPSV23)								
Inactivated poliovirus[7] (IPV)(<18 yrs)			←1st dose→	←2nd dose→	←3rd dose→			
Influenza[8] (IIV; LAIV) 2 doses								

Following the time of young childhood, there's the need for vaccines. This chart outlines that necessity:

18 Months to 18 Years

To get more information regarding the usage of these vaccines, talk to your family doctor. Hepatitis B (HepB) vaccine. (Minimum age: birth)

The routine vaccine at birth

Give one-time HepB vaccine to all infants before discharge from hospital.

If your infant is that were born of hepatitis B antigen surface (HBsAg)-positive mothers, you should administer HepB vaccine as well as 0.5 milliliters hepatitis B immune globulin (HBIG) within 12 hours after the birth. The infants must have a blood test to determine if they are HBsAg, as well as antibodies against the HBsAg (anti-HBs) within 1 to two months following the complete the HepB series, between the ages of 9 to 18 months (preferably during the following well-child appointment).

If the mother's HBsAg level is not known at the time from birth, give HepB vaccine, regardless of weight at birth. Infants who weigh less than 2,000 grams apply HBIG as well as HepB vaccine within 12 hours following the baby's birth. Check the status of mother's HBsAg.

Mayo Clinic Vaccination Schedule, From Birth to 18 Months The Mayo Clinic Schedule of vaccinations is like those in the CDC Schedule above, but may be easier to understand due to the clearness of the written explanations offered through the Clinic. The schedule of vaccinations is created to ensure that children are given vaccinations in the right time in order to safeguard them against illnesses. The schedule is revised every year and the changes can include the introduction of a brand new vaccine, and tweaks to the current recommendations.

Due to the complexity of the schedule as well as the frequent changes The schedule's complexity and frequent updates can make it difficult for parents to keep up-to-date with which vaccinations their children require as well as when. Utilize this checklist to figure the vaccines your child requires right now, and what vaccines will be coming soon according to recommendations from the Centers for Disease Control and Prevention.

If your child suffers from medical issues such as HIV and diabetes or contemplating a trip outside of in the U.S., talk to the doctor to determine if your child should adhere to an alternative schedule of vaccinations.

If your child has missed the dose of vaccine, speak to the doctor to schedule a follow-up vaccine. If you're unsure of what vaccine your child should receive do not hesitate to inquire with your physician. It is also possible to inquire whether you can combine vaccines so that you reduce the amount of shots needed at a single appointment.

Birth

The initial dose of hepatitis B vaccination is typically administered at the time of when you are born. Another dose could be administered at the age of 1 month or after 2 months, when other vaccines are usually offered.

Hepatitis B vaccine, first dose

Age 2 Months

Two months after birth the series of vaccines typically begins. The combination vaccine is generally employed to limit the amount of shots.

Hepatitis B vaccine. 2 doses in case it is not administered at the 1st month

Rotavirus (RV) vaccine, first dose

Tetanus and diphtheria toxoids and Acellular Pertussis (DTaP) vaccination, the first dose

Haemophilus influenzae type b (Hib) conjugate vaccine, first dose

Pneumococcal conjugate vaccine (PCV13), first dose

Inactivated poliovirus vaccine (IPV), first dose

Chapter 9: Reprint From The New York Times

Kate Packard, a school nurse from Seattle is a victim of an unimaginable nightmare that she explains in five words: "measles getting into the water."

If measles does make it to the ferry trip of 20 minutes over Puget Sound from Seattle - it's not impossible, considering the case was discovered in the past near an area of the ferry that is located in West Seattle -- public health officials warn that the entire Vashon School District on the island might be closed down until the case that was last seen on the island went away or until the emergency vaccination campaign took in.

The majority of Vashon Island's 1600 elementary school pupils are legally disinclined to vaccinations against diseases of childhood (2002) that include measles and polio rubella, diphtheria whooping-cough, tetanus the hepatitis B and the chicken pox. It is also a refuge where acupuncture and homeopathy are popular as well as where people complain of health issues among their neighbors kids which they blame on vaccinations.

Many families that opt to skip vaccination have obtained "philosophical exemptions" to the standard vaccine requirements. These exemptions which are available in Washington as well as a few other states, such as California as well as Colorado may be obtained just by signing a school application.

In the United States, approximately 1 percent of the children do not receive vaccination according to the Dr. Walter A. Orenstein director of the National Immunization Program at the Centers for Disease Control and Prevention. Surveys conducted by the agency suggest that over 90 percent of the American children have been given the most vaccinations, with the exception of newly developed chicken-pox vaccination.

From Vashon Island, all the way to Boulder, Colo., to the towns of Missouri and Massachusetts There are hot places" in which a lot of kids are not protected. A survey conducted in 1999 found that eleven states saw increases in the number of exemptions.

Unvaccinated children in clusters could be in threat, officials from the health sector claim, but also pose an attack on the herd immunity" which blocks out outbreaks, securing pregnant women, babies who are too young to receive vaccinations and older people who have weak immune systems and even vaccination-free peers who're still in danger since no vaccine is 100% hundred percent efficient.

In the event that only a small number of parents opt for "herd immunity' for their kids to avoid the tiny risks associated with vaccinations, the system functions.

However, health authorities are worried in states such as California in which it's easy for parents to complete the waiver instead of having their child be vaccinated. The majority of people follow the path of most possible resistance," explained Daniel A. Salmon, an expert on vaccinations in the Johns Hopkins School of Public Health. What I do to my child may make other children more vulnerable." Measles was a problem in 1989 and 1990. out in children of immigrants who were not immunized within Southern California, causing 43,000 cases, and a total of 101 deaths.

The people who are against vaccinations have a variety of justifications. Sometimes, it's a lack of trust in the government officials, believing that they are working with the vaccine industry, and that everyone is making profits from our children", Mr. Salmon said. Some of the concerns are related to religion, like those among Christian Scientists and some Amish groups.

There are times when a group is afraid of a child who is injured by the side effects of the live vaccine against polio, as an example, is believed to result in around 8 deaths per year.

Many parents are irritated by the number of shots that a child needs to receivegenerally around 20 before the age of 2. Some are convinced even though there is evidence that contradicts this that vaccinations have a high chance of causing grave health issues such as seizures or autism.

Health experts from the public sector suggest the resistance to vaccination can be attributed to the efficacy of vaccinations. They say that people are no longer afraid of diseases they've never encountered.

"I can remember how the fear of getting polio affected our lives. We stopped visiting the pool during summer or going to the cinema, and not being engaged in crowds, according to the Dr. Edward P. Rothstein 60 an Pennsylvania pediatrician that helps with the American Academy of Pediatrics make vaccination suggestions. "I can remember images of the wards that were full of iron lung, hundreds of people in one room, and children who were unable to breathe. This affected everyday life more than AIDS can in the present."

With the sporadic adverse effects from the live vaccine an opportunity for about 8 children dying each year (out of millions who were vaccinated) which is why people don't wish to get vaccinated according to him, noting that "when there was a polio outbreak, folks were willing to take the risk."

The Message is Clear

The children and the adults that aren't immunized against most serious diseases place us everyone at danger. This is an issue

It is recommended to be included as a priority for the state legislatures in the states (California, Colorado and Washington among others) providing a fast and straightforward option of being able to "opt-out" of the

The requirement is that children are required to be vaccinated before they can attend the public schools.

Consequences of No Vaccinations

In the past, as hundreds of kids and adults across the United States contracted smallpox, measles, poliomyelitis, or diphtheria each year, security concerns weren't prevalent. There was more fear of the disease itself than any possible adverse effects that could result from the vaccines. Thanks to the popularity of vaccines, the world is a lot different now The diseases are no longer to be feared, and worries concerning the safety of vaccines are frequent.

It is good to know that the majority of parents know benefits of immunizations.

However, it can be difficult for many to recognize the risks which they aren't aware of. In the case of most parents, they aren't aware of an infant paralyzed from the polio virus, or choked to death due to diphtheria or a brain injury caused by measles. In the end, fears of these illnesses does not -- but shouldn't--begin to haunt parents like it did in the past.

It can be difficult to comprehend the significance of vaccines that are new and target ailments that most people aren't aware about, for instance, the vaccine that prevents infection from sexually transmitted human papillomaviruses (HPV). As a 10-year-old one, it's hard to imagine that she is physically active, or the risk of cervical cancer years later since she was never vaccinated for HPV which is a prevalent disease that has no signs.

Although no vaccine is 100 100% safe, dangerous adverse effects are not common. But, since many vaccines are administered to infants in the age range when development or other health issues first start being identified, some parents could believe that vaccines have caused the problem. However, it is challenging to comprehend that the coincidental timing of the vaccine doesn't mean it was the vaccine that caused the issue.

For added stress to make matters worse, media reports of children who's parents think they've been injured by a vaccination which naturally raises concerns for other parents. Then, when parents seek out additional information from the Internet the concerns of parents can get heightened due to the fact that what they discover may appear reasonable, but it could be extremely wrong.